I LOVE A FIRE FIGHTER

I LOVE A FIRE FIGHTER

What the Family Needs to Know

Ellen Kirschman

THE GUILFORD PRESS
New York   London

© 2004 Ellen Kirschman
Published by The Guilford Press
A Division of Guilford Publications, Inc.
370 Seventh Avenue, Suite 1200, New York, NY 10001
www.guilford.com

Printed in the United States of America

This book is printed on acid-free paper.

Last digit is print number: 9   8   7   6

Library of Congress Cataloging-in-Publication Data

Kirschman, Ellen.
  I love a fire fighter : what the family needs to know / by Ellen Kirschman.
      p. cm.
  Includes bibliographical references and index.
  ISBN 978-1-59385-063-0 (pbk.)—ISBN 978-1-59385-084-5 (hardcover)
1. Fire fighters—Job stress. 2. Fire fighters—Family relationships. I. Title.
  HD8039.F5K57 2004
  363.37′01′9—dc22
                                                              2004008303

*This book is dedicated to the men and women
of the fire service and the families who stand with them,
and to my brother, Richard Kirschman,
volunteer fire fighter,
Bolinas Fire Protection District, 1984–2000.
He is the very model of why people love fire fighters.*

Contents

Contents

Acknowledgments

Fire fighters and their families are big-hearted people, enthusiastic about the fire service, and eager to share their experiences. Unfortunately, privacy does not permit me to publicly credit all the individuals, organizations, and departments throughout the United States who opened their doors and welcomed me in.

I am especially grateful to the Greater Cincinnati Fire Media Academy hosted by the Hebron Fire Protection District and organized by fire fighter Mike Fronimos for giving me the hands-on experience to kick-start this project. I also want to acknowledge Chief Ruben Grijalva and the men and women of the Palo Alto Fire Department who have provided me with a professional home for 10 years. They have taught me more than I'll ever teach them.

Many people have contributed to this project by providing information, contacts, feedback, and encouragement. I am grateful to them all, but most especially to my colleagues in public safety psychology: Fire Captain (ret.) Ron Adler; Gary Aumiller, PhD; Carole Ballachey, PhD; Al Benner, PhD; Suzanne Best, PhD; Ann Carr, BS; Burton Clark, PhD; Dave Corey, PhD; Mike Cuttler, PhD; Fire Fighter (ret.) John Durkin, PhD; Gary Fischler, PhD; Doug Gentz, PhD; Richard Gist, PhD; Harvey Goldstein, PhD; Ginger Hayes, PhD; Carl Holmes, EdD; Robin Inwald, PhD; Fire Chief Herb Jewell; Mike Johnson, PhD; Mark Juhas, DSW; Portia Rawles, PsyD; Mike Roberts, PhD; Susan Saxe-Clifford, PhD; Fire Captain Sandy Scheiss; Dave Smith, PhD; Julie Strudlowski,

BA; Phil Trompetter, PhD; Vickie Taylor, LCSW; and Fire Captain (ret.) S. Joseph Woodall. I am especially grateful to Nancy Schwartz and Michael Karter—the good folks at the National Fire Protection Association One Stop Data Shop—for supplying statistics on demand. And I am indebted to my partners at Behaviordyne, William Feister, PhD, and Gary Olson, PhD, for carrying the extra load while I was writing.

I am thankful to the staff at The Guilford Press and to my editor Kathryn Moore for her patience, enthusiasm, and friendship. They are a great crew. Laurie Harper, literary agent, has been generous and supportive. My sister-in-law, Doris Ober, herself a fire fighter spouse, has once again been a literary lifeline. Her skillful editing shows on every page.

I've now written two books about the challenges of living with people in risky occupations. In all fairness, I have to admit that living with a writer is not an easy task either—we are often grumpy, preoccupied, and unavailable. My husband, Steve Johnson, did it cheerfully and patiently. His loving support, kindly wit, and great cooking kept me and the home fires burning.

Preface

This is what I have been waiting for, a live burn. I've worked with fire fighters for many years, but I've never been inside a burning building. So today, after climbing a 100-foot ladder, tearing apart a car with the Jaws of Life, and sitting through hours of classroom lectures about fire behavior, my academy classmates and I are going to suppress our instincts for self-preservation and walk directly into a burning building. I tell myself that as a trained scuba diver, I'm ahead of the game, comfortable with a regulator and an air tank. But it's not the same. It takes me 30 minutes to suit up the first time and I stagger under the heft of nearly 40 pounds of gear. I am festooned with gauges I can't read because my glasses don't fit under my borrowed air mask. I have difficulty hearing my instructors' reassurances about safety because their voices are muffled by my head gear. When I turn to see my reflection in a window, I look more like Paddington Bear than a fire fighter.

As a fire fighter's family member, you'll probably never put on a set of turnouts (protective gear) and walk into a burning building. You may not want to or be allowed to even if you asked. But you are probably very interested in the fire fighter's universe, good and bad, and you may not know where to turn for that information. Unfortunately, many fire departments pay little attention to families, until there is a crisis or someone dies. Even then, information may be scarce.

We walk into the blackened training room: a single, shuffling row of novice fire fighters. I make sure I am last in line so that I am first near the exit. I am sucking air like crazy. Our objective is to understand thermal layering—to experience how heat and smoke rise and why the safest place to be is on the floor where the air is clearest. We are told to kneel, which I do with more than usual effort because of the weight and bulk of my turnouts. It is getting hotter, I feel claustrophobic. My mask seems like it's leaking air, my helmet lists to the left. I am talking to myself, trying to calm myself down. The exit door is as tempting as a chocolate truffle. I am on the verge of panic and struggle to resist the urge to bolt out into the open.

What kind of a job is this, running into buildings normal people are fleeing? What kind of superhuman courage does it take to deliberately, and with full knowledge of the dangers, risk your life for a stranger or a stranger's property? How will my fellow trainees absorb all the required technical and mechanical information they need to stay safe? What about the training required to perform rescues, deal with hazardous materials, and respond to emergency medical calls? Clearly, modern fire science takes more than muscles.

We are now lying on the floor, a daisy chain of prone yellow bodies. The young woman next to me rests her head on my boots and I find her touch strangely comforting. I imagine she is scared and using me as an anchor. This fiction encourages me to maintain my composure for her sake. (When I mention this to her later, she tells me she had no idea where her head was.) It is true, there is more air near the floor and I can see better. The fire has reached the ceiling and is spreading out in all directions. It has a silky, delicate look. Its tendrils are transparent and iridescent, orange in the middle, purple at the edges. It is more beautiful than I had ever imagined. As I watch it burn, I think I understand a tiny bit more about the fascination fire has held for humans throughout history.

Today's fire service is like a world of smoke and mirrors. Things are not always as they seem, and certainly they are not as simple as they once were. The fire service is in the midst of a Herculean struggle to both preserve valued traditions and make necessary changes. This struggle and the ensuing changes affect both fire fighters and their families.

Trying to get a consistent picture of the modern fire service is difficult. While fire fighters share many things in common, there is no prototypical fire fighter and no prototypical fire department. It is as though there are thousands of tiny independent universes. Each department is different, each firehouse is unique, each shift has a personality of its own, and each fire fighter is an individual as well as part of a team. They may all look the same to the public, but their differences are quite apparent to each other and to their families.

It's getting hotter. I'm uncomfortable and have to shift positions. I am determined to stick it out and equally eager to be told to leave. When the order to exit comes, I crawl out, veering sharply away from the door to clear the way for my faster moving classmates. I need a helping hand to stand up. When I turn around, I see my classmates are walking, not crawling, out. I feel humiliated, as though I have exposed the depth of my fear.

Fire fighting is a low-frequency, high-risk business. Most fire fighters spend 80% of their time running medical calls. That's why they train and train and train in these simulated environments. No simulation can ever be perfect because every fire is different and every fireground unique. The key is consistent practice and teamwork. Teamwork is the foundation of a safe, effective operation, and trust is essential to teamwork.

We are preparing to enter the building again. I realize I am wary of my classmates and my instructors alike. I have not had time to build the trust I need to walk back into an inferno, even a controlled one, and I certainly don't trust myself to have the strength or the experience to save my own life. I worry that my companions are so green as to be dangerously overconfident or easily spooked. A story I read recently about a rookie who burned to death in a training fire keeps running through my head.

Fire fighters worldwide regard themselves as a brotherhood. The fire service is built on traditions of service to the community and traditions of mutual support and hospitality to each other. They are a generous group with old-fashioned values. Any day of the year some fire organization will be raising funds for burn victims, sponsoring a toy drive, marching in a parade, or participating in a charitable event. The fire service is a profession where enduring friendships triumph over conflicts; stunning victories trump tragic tales; and acts of selfless courage and heroism overshadow occasional incidents of incompetence or lack of discipline.

I exchange my empty air tank for a full one and walk back into the training tower. I am about to witness a rollover, an intensely hot fire that ignites everything in its path as it satisfies its voracious appetite for oxygen. The temperatures will be close to 1,000 degrees at the ceiling. We are organized in small groups of three. We make our way to an interior room, holding onto the fire hose, which is our lifeline. It is pitch-black. I can't see or hear properly, or feel my way, because I'm completely swathed in heavy gear, with not an inch of exposed skin. My apprehension is high. The instructor orders us to turn around and find our way outside by holding onto the hose line. I have no idea if this is part of the exercise or trouble. Once I hit the outdoors, I decide I've had enough.

ELLEN KIRSCHMAN

I LOVE A FIRE FIGHTER

Introduction

I learned a lot of things in fire school. It was an incredibly enriching and informative experience that expanded my respect for the skill and daring it takes to fight fires, pull bodies from mangled cars, and perform life-saving medical measures in the midst of chaos. It was a powerful adventure fueled by the contagious passion that the students and instructors felt about being fire fighters. Everyone in class wanted to be there and wanted to be successful. Such enthusiasm and dedication is rare in today's workplaces.

Later, as I reviewed the events of the day, something occurred to me. My brother has been a volunteer fire fighter for 16 years. We're very close and talk a lot. I know not to park behind his car in case he's paged away while I'm visiting. Sometimes he even lets me ride along. So, how come, in all these years, he's never told me that the inside of a burning building is pitch-black and fire fighters can't see six inches in front of their faces? When I got home I asked him. He answered that he never mentioned it because it seemed so obvious and he assumed, wrongly as it turns out, that everybody knew this. He didn't want to treat me like a moron or sound like he was pontificating.

This is how it goes for fire fighter families: assumptions are made about what we know or want to know. What's even worse is when other people decide what we *need* to know.

I saw this in the academy. Granted it was a compressed experience—we had a lot to learn in a short period of time. Still, there was not even the briefest mention of fire fighter families or the emotional well-being of fire fighters or how this job may change them and affect their families. No one talked about what it's like to love someone who loves taking risks. No one asked how it feels to be married to a person who is married to his job. No one questioned what fire fighter families need to do to take care of themselves while their mates are away from home taking care of other people. No one acknowledged how the emotional courage fire fighter families need or the independence that is forced on them contributes to the fire service mission. This is extremely puzzling in light of the many studies that confirm how family and friends are the heart of a fire fighter's emotional support system.

Things are changing. In many parts of the country fire fighters' families are starting to insist that their needs be included in fire department protocol. Rookie and veteran families alike are asking to be educated about the psychological and practical implications of being a fire service family. They want recognition and support for their contributions. And they seek reliable, timely information and assistance to sustain themselves during and after emergencies and extended deployments. Families are spearheading this movement because fire fighters' main interests remain directed at issues of physical rather than emotional safety.

This book is intended to bridge the information gap between the fire fighter and his or her family, to raise awareness of the psychological consequences of this work, and to encourage departments to reach out to families. It is my objective to describe the subtle and obvious ways the demands of this unique occupation spill over to home and to suggest strategies that families—meaning parents, children, siblings, spouses, friends, and significant others—can use to manage the spillover and/or learn to live with it.

In many ways this is also a book about change in a culture that values tradition. In this post-9/11 world, fire fighters and their families have serious new worries about health and safety along with more familiar worries. I try to address some of these concerns by looking at the physical and emotional dangers of this profession and the amazing progress that has been made to bolster fire fighter safety.

While fire fighters have an almost mythical status in our society, their families see them in a more realistic light. It is from that perspective that I describe the positive and negative attributes of people who want to be fire fighters, what it's like to live with them, and how they may change over time. I also consider how they are affected by work-related organizational stress and line-of-duty trauma, and how these changes may affect their relationships. When trouble strikes, I have suggestions about what families can do to help their mates, their children, and themselves, and where they can turn for help.

To the best of my ability I've tried to represent the experiences of both career and volunteer fire fighters. There's a lot of overlap between these two groups. Many paid fire fighters are volunteers in their spare time and many volunteers are seeking work in the career service. While there are differences, sometimes profound ones, between the two groups, studies suggest they share similar dispositions. Both enjoy other people's company, are open to new experiences, like excitement and activity, are concerned for the welfare of others, and want to help people in need.

Because the fire service is so large and complex, I've had to make some hard choices. Unfortunately, there are not enough pages in this book to give wildland fire fighters, arson investigators, search and rescue teams, hazardous materials teams, bomb squads, high angle and water rescue teams, and others the attention they truly deserve.

Dr. Carl Holmes, retired assistant chief of the Oklahoma City Fire Department, travels a lot and likes to tell people that no matter what city he's in, when he eats at McDonald's, he gets the exact same number of french fries with every order. "Why," he asks his listeners, "can McDonald's pay employees six dollars an hour and get consistency in their products, and the fire service can't hardly get consistency between shifts?" He exaggerates for effect, but his message is on point. There is great diversity of practice in the U.S. fire service. Most of the departments I visited and studied and the people I met were highly professional and progressive in their management of both technical and human resources. Others were less so, and some seemed truly behind the times. I have drawn stories from the entire range. Consequently, as you read this book you might find yourself thinking "That's not the way it is here" as often as you think "That sounds just like us."

The same is true for stories I tell about families and individuals. While there is a range of difficulties shared by fire fighters and their families, the clear majority of those I met seem truly content with their lives. My emphasis on the "hot spots"—and I found some—should not be generalized to the entire fire service or understood as a prediction of things to come. Look at it this way: some of the more troubling issues will apply to you or to people you know only some of the time. But, as a psychologist, I know that when and if troubled times come, it makes matters worse to be blindsided by the unexpected. People who are informed and prepared in advance remain calmer under stress and are more effective problem solvers.

The anecdotes in this book were gathered from interviews I collected all over the United States and from the files of my colleagues. Some examples are composites. Except when expressly permitted, all names and identifying information have been disguised. Fire fighters and their families are very generous people and everyone I spoke to gave me permission to use their names and their stories. It was my decision to keep most anecdotes anonymous.

Feel free to use this book like a medical manual, turning to the chapters that are most relevant to you and your family. Some chapters or parts of chapters may seem weighted more toward the family than the fire fighter or vice versa, as might the tips that follow most chapters. My hope is that *all* the material will be of interest and benefit to every reader—fire fighter and family member alike.

CHAPTER 1

Beepers in Your Bedroom

The Givens and Realities of the Fire Service

Certain challenges face fire fighters and their families. Some of these are not unique to the fire service or even to other emergency responders. This is a paradox. On the one hand, fire fighters and their families occupy a special place in society. On the other hand, it is too limiting and isolating to say that no one else understands their challenges. Despite widespread use of easy slogans about the sanctity of family life and family values, our society does too little to support working families in many occupations.

When I interviewed fire fighters and their families I tried to identify themes that came up repeatedly. I called these themes "givens" because they are aspects of the fire service that probably won't ever change much. The first is learning to share your loved one with the *firehouse family*. The second is dealing with *shift work and separations*. The third is coping with *long hours* at work. The fourth is dealing with *unpredictable schedules and emergencies*. The fifth is *worry*. And the sixth is living with *public scrutiny*.

THE FIREHOUSE FAMILY: MARRIED TO THE JOB

Maybe it's my age, maybe it's my gender, but a lot of what occurs in the fire service seems to me to have something to do with the way men relate to one another and how they behave in groups. This is similar to the behavior observed in other mostly male occupations like the military, athletics, the construction trades, and so on. (Even women fire fighters show some of these traits as they try to fit into work cultures designed by men.)

Obviously there are good and bad aspects to this bonding—as you'll learn from the following stories—but the good seems to outweigh the bad. Real families are usually reluctant to share their fire fighter with his or her firehouse family, but, as I discovered, most do eventually grow accustomed to this dual allegiance and some even learn to use it their advantage. On the positive side, being part of the firehouse family almost guarantees that you will have a safety net in times of crisis. Fire fighters are great at providing social and practical support to each other's families. Belonging to the firehouse family also means you get to share in the pride of being part of an elite and esteemed profession. You will have the respect and admiration of your community, and your children will get the same respect and admiration from their peers.

In the beginning, it takes some getting used to the fact that fire fighters consider the fire service their second family but sometimes behave as though it is their first. Career and volunteer fire fighters alike describe the fire station as a place to hang out, rest up from their "real jobs," escape from their "real families," and avoid the "honey do" list waiting for them at home. They say this only half in jest. It is clear that for some the firehouse is a male sanctuary in peril of disappearing as women join the fire service: a place where "boys can be boys," tell crude jokes, and play with trucks and tools.

Take a look into one urban firehouse in the Northeast. It's shift change and there are a lot of fire fighters milling around, some getting ready to leave, others just coming in. Pete grabs a cup of coffee and throws himself in a lounge chair feigning utter exhaustion. "I need a rest," he says. "My wife has been running me ragged. The only time I get to sit down is when I'm working."

Pete has an electrical contracting business, three small children, and a wife who loves to garden. When he's home it's nonstop activity. By comparison, work as a fire fighter is a breeze and he refers to it as his "part-time job."

"Listen up, Lenny, you can still change your mind," someone says to a recently engaged fire fighter.

"Hey, leave him alone, he's still in lust," shouts Pete.

"Yo, Lenny," someone else chimes in. "Do you know the best way to cure a nymphomaniac? Marry her!"

Everyone in the room laughs. They've all heard it before and it still strikes them as funny. This is the warm-up, a time to check each other out. Who's in a good mood, who had a foul four days off? Gauging each other's mood is important; these guys are going to be together for the rest of the shift. Working fire fighters never go anywhere alone: when one goes, they all go. When they shop for lunch and dinner, they travel in pods chained together by possibility, ready to spring into action if and when they are dispatched to a call. Living, training, eating, risking, and relaxing on and off duty with the same group of people year in and year out breeds an intimacy that comes close to the intimacy one usually shares with real family. After a while everybody knows everybody's moods and personal habits.

There are major benefits to being part of such a close and often closed community, one that has it's own values, rituals, norms, language, and humor. For one thing, it's a very powerful support system and consequently a robust buffer against stress. One study of 1,700 fire fighters and fire fighter/paramedics concluded that even though at-home social support was more highly rated than at-work support, at-work social support had a more positive influence on job satisfaction, the perception of occupational stress, and stress-related health outcomes. This is because at-work support is more immediate, more timely, and more relevant. When a fellow fire fighter/paramedic says you've done a good job, the presumption is that he or she really knows what a "good job" is.

Part of the price of belonging to this family is a shift in identity from "me" to "we," the same shift that needs to happen in a good marriage or any other significant relationship. That means most fire fighters have dual allegiances. It can be stressful trying to be loyal to two families and to fill two roles like fire fighter and parent. On the other hand, current research suggests that multiple roles are actually beneficial to mental, physical, and relationship health. Look at these documented findings on multiple roles:

- The negatives and dissatisfactions of one role are buffered by the positives and satisfactions of another role.
- There are increased opportunities for social support. People who have extensive on-the-job networks are more satisfied with their family life and childcare arrangements, plus their children are healthier and do better in school.
- There are increased opportunities to experience success.
- There are expanded opportunities to see things from different perspectives and receive feedback from varied sources.
- A person's sense of self can broaden and become more multidimensional.
- Flexible gender roles can lead to more closeness, sharing, and friendship between partners, especially those with children.
- Workers who are married with children have more family-to-work conflict than single or childless workers, but their family life has far more positive effects on their work. Support from home helps them deal with work problems and feel more confident.

The challenge for fire fighter families is to figure out how to reap the benefits of their multiple roles. Annual social events at the firehouse do not come close to providing families with the same level of camaraderie and support that fire fighters get, or that their families say they want. Families need to get together with each other and also be included in departmental activities like trainings, briefings, and wellness programs.

Learning to Play Second Fiddle

Real fire fighter families commonly feel as though they play second fiddle to the work family. It's easy to see how this happens. Who wouldn't feel abandoned when her or his fire fighter spouse leaps up in the middle of dinner to respond to a call, has to work during important family events, has a second job to support his chosen first job, gets in a minor accident with you in the car and seems more concerned about the other driver's injuries than yours, or spends what little time she has at home listening to the scanner? Take heart, you may not always feel this way. Many spouses report that life is hardest in the beginning, especially with small children to raise. Ultimately they grow accustomed to the schedules and the separations, even the fear, because they have to. Among other things, pride in their mates' devotion to helping others makes it easier to cope with loneliness, anxiety, and resentment.

Rachel began dating Mark, a volunteer fire fighter, when they were both in their mid-thirties. She'd never known a fire fighter before. Each of them had been divorced, so they were taking things slowly. Mark was especially cautious about revealing the depths of his feelings. The first time he dared tell Rachel he loved her they were lying in bed. No sooner did he declare his love than the alarm went off and he scrambled into his clothes and flew out the door. He came back in an hour, apologized for his abrupt departure, took off his clothes, and climbed back into bed, reassuring Rachel that such late-night interruptions were rare. As soon as he lay down, the alarm went off again, and once more he dashed out the door. When he came home after the third alarm, Rachel was seriously doubting that this was the life for her.

At the time Rachel thought she would never get used to Mark going out and leaving her alone in the middle of the night. She found it especially difficult during this early "romantic" period. Twenty years later, he wakes her up while getting into bed and she asks him if he's just been to the bathroom—only to learn that he's been out of the house for six hours!

Mark is now a career fire fighter and deputy chief of operations. Rachel still doesn't like it when his pager goes off in the middle of the night because she doesn't easily fall back to sleep when he's out on a call. It's not that she's afraid: she knows his job is to run the scene, not to run into the fire. But she hates getting comfy in bed expecting him to be home as planned at 11:00 P.M., only to have him call and say he won't be there until 1:00 A.M. When he does come in around 2:00 A.M., he wakes her out of a sound sleep. What helps is that Rachel recognized early on that the qualities she loves about Mark are the same attributes that

9

made him want to be a fire fighter: his desire to help and his sensitivity to others.

It's inevitable: in some ways, and at some times, you are going to feel as if your mate loves his or her job more than he or she loves you. Ironically, the dedication, commitment, and pride that are so much a part of the tradition and culture of the fire service may be the very things that irritate and alienate fire fighter families. Being a fire fighter is not just a job, it's an identity, a beloved hobby, and, for good and bad, a second family. That doesn't mean that fire fighters don't have room to love their real families, but it does mean that your relationship can feel a little crowded. You need plenty of self-worth and independence to share so much of your life. A sense of humor also helps.

Rita Brunacini, wife of Alan Brunicini, chief of the Phoenix, Arizona fire department, was having one of those days when she was feeling like a second fiddle. She was angry and confronted her husband. "I think you love Fire Station 1 more than you love me," she complained. "Yes, I do," he admitted, "but I love you more than Fire Station 2."

It sounds strange, but it can be liberating to come to terms with the fact that your mate is crazy about fire paraphernalia and always will be. You don't have to love fire trucks yourself, but it helps to make an effort to share and understand the commitment and pride that your fire fighter feels about his or her chosen profession.

Every family is different and every family has to figure out how best to live with this profession. There is no formula, no right or wrong way.

Elaine told me flat out, "When I got married, I married my husband's department too and expanded my dysfunctional family by 46 people!" She was only half joking about the dysfunctional part. She would never make her husband choose between her and his job, so she settled in and got involved. Her advice to new spouses? "If you're not already independent, you need to learn how to be." Elaine is very clear that when she chose to marry a fire fighter, she also chose the lifestyle that came with him—a choice she has had to remake over and over as the years passed. She has a great sense of humor. "Forget about competing with the department," she says, "lights and sirens win out over sexy lingerie every time!"

Accepting the firehouse family as part of the package is one approach, especially if the person you marry is already a fire fighter. But what happens if you marry a teacher and two years later he decides to join the fire service? Amy was pretty miserable when Lee made his decision. She hated being alone so much of the time, even though she needed the time to study. She worried about Lee's safety. She trusted him, but she didn't much like it that there were female fire fighters sleeping in his dorm. Amy's attitude changed when there was a small fire at their house. Fire fighters came from all over, from as far away as 30 miles. She remembers that "fire fighters were literally running people off the road to get to us just because we're part of the family." As she tells me this story, she has tears in her eyes.

It's a great anecdote, but I wondered why it took a crisis for Amy to feel welcomed and supported by Lee's department. Shouldn't she have been included as a valued part of the fire service from the beginning? Where were the people who could have talked to her about everyday concerns like coping with loneliness? Who could have eased her fears about Lee's safety? Unfortunately, spousal support programs are few and far between. Those that exist are found mostly in large urban fire departments.

Amy's experience as a fire victim reveals the depths of the commitment fire fighters have to one another and the benefits of being part of the fire service. Here are three more examples out of dozens I collected.

When Angel's whole family was hospitalized with a mystery virus, his coworkers called everyday. "It's amazing," he says. "It doesn't make any difference if people like me or not, they'll come to help."

Cindy used to make fun of her husband, Dave, and imitate him talking on his radio in front of their family. When her mother had a heart attack, fire fighter/paramedics arrived in a flash, saved her life, and were very supportive in the process. Cindy's sister was staying with their mother. She was so grateful that she called Cindy and told her she'd hit her if she ever mocked Dave again.

Laci and Evan have four children. Evan is in the National Guard and he was deployed overseas for six months. While he was gone Laci made a decision not to share any bad news from home with him. She wanted Evan to stay focused on what he was doing and not worry about the family, especially since there was little he could do from so far away. She didn't tell him when their health insurance lapsed and their youngest son needed surgery. But the fire department knew and took up a collection to pay for the surgery. When Laci declares that "I'm not just married to a fire fighter, I'm married to the whole fire fighter family," she says so not with resentment, but with pride, gratitude, and the certain knowledge that she can depend on Evan's department in times of need.

MANAGING SHIFT WORK AND SEPARATIONS

Separations are part and parcel of the emergency response life-style. There's a high likelihood that your fire fighter will be working at night, on holidays, on your birthday, on your child's birthday, when the pipes burst, and when the dog has puppies. Fire fighters can be called in or called back just as guests are arriving for dinner or just when you were counting on leaving the kids at home and getting away for the day.

That's what happened to Mindy. She was on her shift when the dog bit her son in the face. Her partner, Morgan, called from the hospital hysterical and crying. Mindy told her captain to find backup and literally flew out the door. Home was two hours away. By the time she got to the hospital she was almost in hysterics herself. She "did an O.J." through the parking lot toward the emergency room (ER) doors, which opened outward, knocking her flat on her butt. By the time she found Morgan, their son was in surgery. Morgan was furious with her for days. It didn't make any difference that Mindy drove like lightning and ran like the wind: she wasn't there when she was needed. Morgan's anger was irrational; Mindy might not have been home if she sold insurance. It was just his wife's cumulative total of spending time away from home that got to Morgan who was feeling, for the moment, consumed with responsibility and worry.

There are a variety of work schedules in the career fire service ranging from 9- to 24-hour shifts. Each schedule has its plusses and minuses in terms of sleeping, eating, commuting, and time off. One thing is sure: shift work can make life difficult, especially when you're trying to keep little children quiet so that Mom or Dad can sleep during the day. Your family, your non-fire service friends, and your children's schoolteachers may all be affected by your fire fighter's schedule and be upset when he or she isn't predictably available or can't be counted on to show up and stay as planned.

On the other hand, there are many positives associated with shift work. For one thing, it gives parents the opportunity to spend more time with their children than they might on a regular 9:00–5:00 schedule. And, according to recent studies, the more a man is involved in childcare, the better his psychological well-being and the better his wife feels about their marriage. This is why it's important to share both information and discipline. Protecting your mate from bad news that occurred when he was working can make him feel like an uninformed outsider. Likewise, telling your kids to "wait until your father gets home" can set him up as the "house heavy."

Here's a partial list of what some spouses have learned to like about shift work. It's also a great example of the value of focusing on the positive rather than on the negative. See if you can add to this list. Post it where you can use it as a reminder when and if you're feeling down.

- "A little breathing space."
- "Privacy, peace, and quiet."
- "One-on-one time alone with children, my friends, or family."
- "I get to have the whole bed to myself."
- "Time to do my own thing."
- "Help with childcare and sick kids."
- "Someone to pick the kids up at school and be there when they get home."
- "Time to simmer down when I'm mad."
- "I know where he is and what he's doing. If he was going to a bar every third night, I'd be jealous."

Sometimes separations can be extensive. Wildland fire fighters and search and rescue teams, for example, are often deployed elsewhere for weeks and months at a time. And all fire fighters can be called back for an emergency or pressed into service when mutual aid is required. Lilly's husband, Mel, a fire fighter/paramedic, was once again deployed to a major wildfire. It was a dangerous assignment: the winds were fierce and the fire was out of control. Lilly's kids were watching the fire on TV when they saw Mel. "Dad's on TV!" they yelled. Lilly couldn't bear to look. She asked the kids, "Is he on a stretcher?" When the answer was "No," she went back to what she was doing.

Lilly has grown used to Mel being gone during wildland fire season; there have been three or four occasions when he has been deployed out of state for weeks at a time. Any big fire in the western United States means he might be called away. It was hard when their children were small—he was away when their youngest broke his foot—and harder still being both Mom and Dad to teenagers. But they got through it all because they have a strong family support system and deeply held religious beliefs. They have also learned to prepare themselves and their children for these separations and to lower their expectations for reunions. When Mel comes home they take things slowly and know it will be awhile before things return to normal. No one taught Lilly and her children how to steel themselves for these separations: they learned "on the job." As a result, Mel and Lilly's children are flexible, independent, responsible, and community-minded.

Long separations present challenges, particularly at homecoming. People change, expectations differ. Families of a local urban search and rescue team that went to Oklahoma City in response to the Murrah building bombing were expecting to spend time together catching up and reestablishing intimacy. Instead, their loved ones spent most of the first few days at home talking to the media, giving speeches, and accepting awards. The primary way families learned anything about the deployment was by watching TV news or listening to their fire fighters talking on the telephone to other fire fighters. Children were sulky, distant, or clingy. Couples felt awkward with one another. In some families there was competition over who had it worse during their time apart. Many families felt that their fire fighters didn't have a clue about what it took to "hold down the fort" and wished they had been recognized in ceremonies honoring the returning "heroes." Getting back to normal took longer than expected.

Families fared better in another part of the country where spouses organized a program for families affected by the deployment. They set up predeployment workshops so veteran spouses could tell new families what it was like to be alone and what they needed to do to keep their families together. It was a time to prepare psychologically for the long separation and for the "after-action stress" brought on by the media deluge, the public adoration, and the persistent feelings of being left out. This group set up an 800 number for families to call for updates and made sure that the department issued timely information about the deployment. They held family briefings during and after the deployment, and lobbied for including families in public events and ceremonies.

LIVING WITH LONG HOURS

Hank is a captain, or company officer. Since he's been promoted he works 56 or more hours a week including his days off. There is always someplace he has to go, a last-minute meeting, or training. He spends a lot more time at work than he did when he worked as a computer technician. He gets paid for overtime, but he still takes offense that people think fire fighters have so much time off.

His long hours are a problem for his wife, Nancy. The kids drive her nuts and she feels like a "single parent" with two incomes. Hank recognizes that she has a lot to handle and that their family life is very different from the one she grew up in. He knows she gets mad, but he also knows that she usually gets over it the next day. While he's sympathetic, he also sounds irritated. He and Nancy met when he was a line fire fighter, and he thinks she should have known how their life together would be. Unfortunately, what you expect and how it actually feels can be quite different.

Hank wishes that Nancy understood that he would rather be at home. He misses his children a lot and knows they miss him. He looks like he's enjoying himself at work—who wants to be a grouch?—but underneath he feels sad. His daughter cries for him at bedtime. He may be gone just one 24-hour shift, but to a small child that's a lifetime. Young children, especially, need quality *and* quantity time with parents. It's hard for Hank's daughter to warm up to him when he's been gone for a day. She's not old enough to soothe her disappointment at not seeing him. He knows this and regularly telephones home at bedtime. This helps, but it's not the same as being there to tuck her in.

Besides working as a paid fire fighter, Hank volunteers three to four hours a week for his local fire department. He's convinced that if he didn't there wouldn't be enough volunteers. Hard to tell, but I suspect "being needed" as a supervisor and a volunteer is the way Hank rationalizes overriding Nancy's objections and doing what he wants to do. This is a choice he's making. I hope he's prepared for the consequences for him and for his marriage. I also hope that Nancy has friends and family to support her and that ultimately they acheive greater balance between work and family.

On the other hand, maybe Hank is truly burdened by divided loyalties and a heavy sense of responsibility. He admits that many of his fire fighter friends have been divorced because they committed too much time to the job, but he apparently doesn't think this will happen to him. Nancy wishes Hank worried about her as much as he worries about his crew. He says he does, but it apparently doesn't feel that way to her. This is something they should be talking about, but first they have to find the time.

THE FOURTH ALARM: UNPREDICTABILITY AND EMERGENCIES

All emergency responders are subject to being called up, called back, or delayed without notice. Volunteers never know when they will be needed and career fire fighters can catch a bad fire late in their shift, delaying their return home. Catastrophes, disasters, and major incidents all happen without warning and without any regard for the plans you may have made.

Jack was almost late to his own wedding. He is so proud of being a fire fighter that he was determined to borrow a fire truck to drive to the church for the afternoon ceremony. He was waxing the truck when a structure fire call came in. It took three hours to knock the fire down. Then he had to wash and wax the truck all over again because it was filthy. Four of the men in his wedding were on the call with him and they were also delayed. Jack and his friends got to the church an hour late. His fiancée, Jenny, was frantic and angry. It wasn't a great beginning to their marriage—although it was a sample of their future life together.

Jack would miss a lot of "firsts": his son's first birthday, first Thanksgiving, and first Christmas. On their first Valentine's Day as a married couple, Jenny made a special romantic dinner that went uneaten when Jack was called out on an emergency. She was very disappointed and his in-laws were incensed when they heard about it. Jack's in-laws think it is the height of rudeness to leave the dinner table before the meal is over, even though Jack's leaving had absolutely nothing to do with manners and everything to do with duty and a huge fire. Jenny's parents' reaction caused a lot of friction at home. Ultimately Jenny had to, in Jack's words, "Tell her parents to mind their own business."

Jenny has gotten better at changing her plans on a moment's notice. She's less needy than she was as a young mother, and today she doesn't require so much attention from Jack. Now that their kids are older she enjoys the time she has to herself. She hasn't forgotten how hard it once was, but now the memories make her laugh. She can remember planning a boating trip with Jack and the children. His pager went off and the next thing she saw was their truck with the boat still attached speeding down the road. She and the kids stood in the driveway crying, surrounded by picnic baskets and fishing gear. It was hours before she found out where he had gone, and by then she was absolutely furious.

It was this incident that helped Jack and Jenny see that they needed more balance in their family life. Jack understood that he needed to be more considerate, and Jenny learned that she needed to be more flexible. While cell phones and pagers helped a lot, they both prefer more old-fashioned ways to stay in touch. Jack writes his schedule on a family calendar that his kids can understand and he leaves greeting cards, surprise Post-it notes, and special treats in his children's lunchboxes on the days he's working.

Planned outings can be rescheduled and holiday celebrations can be postponed, but one-time-only events like dance recitals and athletic competitions cannot. When Jack couldn't swing a tour trade to attend his daughter's school play, he made sure she knew, in advance, how much he would miss being there. He showed as much interest as possible—went to rehearsals, helped build the stage set, and arranged for Jenny to videotape the event.

On the day of the play he left his daughter a note wishing her luck and sent flowers later. The next day they watched the video together and talked in detail about how things went.

When disaster strikes, Jack, Hank, and all their fellow fire fighters have a responsibility to their community. Those on duty will be expected to stay for their entire shift and may even be held over. Those at home will be expected to leave their homes and respond to where they are needed, which may be miles away. In large emergencies you may not know where your mate has been deployed or when he or she is expected home. Watching TV news may give you some information, but it will also raise your anxiety, especially if there is word of fire fighters being injured or killed. Families should never get bad news over the TV or the radio. Unfortunately, it sometimes happens that way.

On the opposite end, your fire fighter may be consumed with worry about your welfare and the welfare of your children and your home. He may feel awful knowing that you are anxious about him. She may be terribly upset at not being able to call home and reassure you that she is okay. These kinds of concerns can interfere with concentration and safety.

Joanie and Haps have worked out a system that's carried them through the past 10 years. They each carry digital pagers and have worked out identifying call signs and codes conveying degrees of urgency from "Call when you can" to "Call now—all hell has broken loose!" Like most fire fighter families, they are self-taught, industrial-strength copers, who learned as they went along.

Fire fighter families have a lot to be proud of. Most have spent years pinch-hitting for their absent fire fighters and handling tough times alone. They have built-in shock absorbers and manage to keep their families on track even when their lives are turned upside-down by the unexpected.

Bill injured his knee playing in the annual police versus fire fighters football game. He was out of work for six long months. His injury was not job-related, so he had almost no money coming in to support his four small children and his wife, Edie, who was a full-time mother. When Bill's brother, a real estate broker, offered Edie a temporary job filling in as his office manager, she took it and Bill watched the kids. It was an interesting switch with an unexpected benefit. Edie liked working so much that when Bill returned to his job, she went back to school and got her real estate license.

WORRY: MANAGING YOUR ANXIETY

Fire fighting is sometimes seen as more stressful and dangerous by families than by fire fighters themselves. TV dramas and so-called reality shows that routinely feature plot lines in which there is no downtime or boredom—only countless crises, relentless danger, and endless acts of superhuman heroism—amplify these perceptions. And, of course, the events of September 11th reinforced and fortified everyone's fears.

Families don't have the benefit of training, and most of all they lack the kind of encouragement and reassurance their loved ones get at the fire station. Belonging to the firehouse family reinforces fire fighters' sense of control over the environment and over their work. As they experience excitement and exhilaration on the job, it tends to increase their self-esteem and balance the apprehension they may feel while doing dangerous work.

Much of the downtime in firehouses is spent telling stories—stories that one psychologist compared to medieval epics because they had staying power: fires in the distant past are written about and spoken of as though they happened yesterday. These stories often emphasize values such as courage, loyalty, and valor. They instill a sense of tradition as well as expectations for the future. As a consequence, they amplify and enhance both self-esteem and job satisfaction by reinforcing the prestige and uniqueness of belonging to an elite culture.

Families don't get to share in these antidotes against worry—which is one of the reasons I wrote this book. It would also help if departments sponsored educational and social events where families could ask questions, express concerns, and network with each other (see end-of-chapter Tips). These events or parts of them might best be closed to fire fighters in order to eliminate the possibility of family members being "coached" not to ask "embarrassing" questions.

The bottom line is that people do learn to live with worry,

and often they do it in their own unique ways. Pat Brandt, a nurse and fire fighter wife, told interviewer Samantha Dunn that she has gone through four stages in her marriage. She called the first stage "ignorance" and said she really didn't want to know what her husband did at work. Shortly thereafter she moved to the second stage, "preoccupation," when she bought a scanner and listened to it all the time. It kept her in a constant state of anxiety. One day she showed up at the scene of a dangerous call she heard on the scanner. The following morning when her husband came home he threw the scanner at the living room wall and broke it beyond repair.

The third stage was a short period of "denial" during which Pat refused to talk to her husband about his work. This ultimately made them feel like strangers and Pat moved to her fourth, and hopefully final, stage, "accepting concern." She doesn't seek out bad news, but she lets her husband know that she is and will be available to listen.

PUBLIC SCRUTINY: SHARING THE HEAT

There are times when fire fighters get bad press. It's very painful to read negative things about the person you love or about his or her chosen profession. When a fire fighter sets a fire, steals money, assaults a coworker, or seduces a fellow fire fighter's widow, it makes headlines. That doesn't happen as consistently for other occupations, except police. Fire fighters and fire fighters' families were outraged when the author of a book about the destruction of the World Trade Center implied that a company of fallen fire fighters had secreted stolen merchandise in their fire truck before dying and that others, working rescue and recovery, were guilty of stealing laptops and purses from damaged buildings.

Fire fighters are often public scapegoats, taking the heat for a catastrophe. After the Oakland Hills fire that destroyed 3,500 dwellings and killed 25 people, some residents who intentionally chose to live in the woodsy, fire-prone hills seemed more intent on blaming their losses on the fire department than assuming responsibility themselves. It was a frightening and tragic fire with many mistakes and much more heroism.

Human beings are meaning-making animals. We need to know why things happen as they do. In the aftermath of tragedy, particularly one that might have been avoided or lessened, we want to identify villains and assign blame. Complex situations get oversimplified. Revenge and reasonable needs for accountability blur. All this can be hell on families who know how hard fire fighters work and how much they care.

It's not always tragedy that brings public scrutiny. Fire fighters attract negative as well as positive stereotypes. They can be seen as hard-drinking, lazy, and egotistical. When the economy is bad, their day-to-day activities come under scrutiny and are weighed in terms of worth to the community. Such public debate, while necessary, is exceptionally painful to fire fighters and their families. Fire fighters have been told to keep firehouse apparatus doors closed even on the hottest nights so that taxpayers won't see them sitting around waiting for the alarm to go off. It's a wild oscillation to go from being heroes to being bad guys: one day everyone thinks you're wonderful and the next day they're accusing you of feeding at the public trough. Bad jokes, hate mail, angry editorials, and snide comments can replace the cards and the cookies in the blink of an eye. Sometimes it's even hard to read positive press. Many families of New York City fire fighters resented the hero image attributed to their spouses in the days after 9/11. They feared that making heroes out of their husbands simply set them up for further danger because heroes don't have human limits.

Tips for Dealing with the Givens

- Work out some "homecoming" habits. Homecoming is the "arsenic hour"—everyone has needs and no one has anything left to give. Everyone unwinds differently. Many emergency responders want a break from problems before tackling family concerns. Learn about each other's needs. Respect your differences.

(cont.)

(continued from previous page)

- It helps to give each other a brief summary of the ups and downs of what's happened since you last saw each other. If your mate is grouchy, at least you'll know why.
- Make dates with each other and write them down on a family calendar. Knowing you will have some time alone with each other may be what gets you through the week. It's harder to act spontaneously than to break a planned date. When you do get time to yourselves, turn off the pager and the TV and don't answer the telephone.
- Introduce your children to the firehouse as early as possible. Include them in social events. Let them play with the equipment. Buy them books and toys related to fire fighting. Do what you can to help them form a mental picture of what Mom or Dad is doing when she or he is away from home. This may help young children in particular to stay emotionally connected to a physically absent parent.
- Children are extremely proud of their fire-fighting parents. This eases their dissapointment when Mom or Dad has to work and miss a special occasion. Reinforce this pride by attending school and social events in uniform, participating in career days, talking about your work at home, and so on.
- Create your own family rituals and holiday celebrations. Explore your family heritage for ideas.
- If shift work is negatively affecting your sex life, talk about it. Try making dates to have sex rather than waiting to be "in the mood." You can't force yourself to feel sexy, but scheduling may help make it a priority. So might strategically placed, intimate Post-it notes.
- Make the most of the time you have together. Turn everyday chores—a trip to the supermarket or the recycling center, for example—into a family outing. Exercise together, perform community service as a family, turn off the TV, and play games.
- Insist that your mate deal with you and not use the job as a scapegoat or a way to avoid confronting problems.
- Many career fire fighters work second jobs to supplement their pay. Working long hours to support a family who never

sees you should prompt you to reevaluate your finances and your priorities.

- Make decisions about optional career choices—promotions, speciality assignments, and so on—as a family. After all, these kinds of decisions affect everyone in the family and everyone in the family will be pressed to support them.
- Work out a system of "rainchecks." Treat yourselves to something special when your plans are canceled at the last minute. Sometimes just planning a special outing can take the edge off mutual disappointment.
- Monitor your own and your children's TV viewing, particularly during a crisis involving fire fighters.
- Keep things in perspective. Try not to take bad press personally. Neither of you is responsible for apologizing for or explaining the fire service's actions. It is okay to say "I don't know" or "I don't want to talk about this this now." Prepare in advance to deal with intrusive or critical comments.
- Turnaround is fair play. Consider arranging for your spouse to have 24 hours of getaway time to rest and rejuvenate.
- Dare to go places by yourself rather than miss out on things that are important to you. The awkwardness will become a thing of the past with practice. Use your time alone to advantage. Think about what stimulates and gratifies you intellectually, emotionally, spiritually, and physically. Plan ahead for times you know you'll be alone.
- If you're scared to be home alone, say so. You have every right to feel comfortable and safe. Consider installing a security alarm, motion detector lights, and security locks on the windows and doors. Get a dog.
- Find other fire fighter spouses and families who will be alone at night or on holidays. Get together with them. Share childcare.
- Don't try to change your fire fighter or get him or her to quit. Once a fire fighter, always a fire fighter. Your other options? Choose to be part of their lives and risk taking time from your own interests. Or choose to make your own life and risk drifting apart. Everyone is different. There are no perfect

(*cont.*)

(continued from previous page)

"one-size-fits-all" solutions. Aim for arrangements that work 85% of the time and forget the other 15%.

- Pour your heart out on an online message board or in a chat room for fire fighter families (see Resources). They'll understand.
- Become as self-sufficient as possible. Learn how to do basic home repairs and prepare your home for emergencies (see Resources).
- Attend spouses' academies. If there isn't an academy in your department or your district, talk to someone about starting one. A spousal academy should include:
  - Identifying job-related stressors
  - Recognizing the signs and symptoms of acute and cumulative stress
  - Understanding the changes that fire fighters and emergency medical personnel undergo
  - Defining how job-related stress can spill over to the family and how family stress can spill over to the job
  - Providing information about job benefits, including programs that offer counseling, fitness advice, chaplains' services, and critical incident debriefings
- Consider putting together a spousal support program, ideally with department support. Consult the Resources for assistance. A support program might consist of:
  - A family needs assessment
  - Advocacy for family needs
  - Including family members in peer support programs
  - Special family debriefings for extended incidents, red alerts, bioterrorism, and so on.
  - A telephone tree and/or e-mail list
  - A family section on the department website
  - Participation in/observation of fire fighter training
  - Participation in health and wellness programs

CHAPTER **2**

Spillover
Managing the Relationship
between Home and Work

Fire fighters live in two separate worlds, home and work, each requiring a different set of social skills. There is plenty of positive overlap, but sometimes what works well in one place may not be appreciated or helpful in the other. Considering these things in advance gives you a head start on dealing with them, if and when they spill over to your family. Are these issues exclusive to fire fighter families? I doubt it. Are they common in the fire service? I think so.

COMMUNICATION PROBLEMS

One of the most common complaints families make is about lack of communication. One of the most common dillemmas fire fighters have is how much to tell. Every individual and every couple is unique. Some spouses, like Betsy, have absolutely no interest in the fire service beyond remembering that her husband works every third day and gets paid every other Friday.

Stell's needs are different and she's extremely frustrated with her husband, Rand. Rand was responsible for coordinating ground rescue at the site of a commercial airline disaster. There were body parts everywhere. The magnitude of the carnage was so extreme that normally stoic, experienced personnel were overwhelmed and had to be removed from the scene.

Rand's duties kept him on-site for days. When he came home, Stell asked him repeatedly how he was. He answered, "I'm okay," to which she would reply, "You can't be okay—talk to me." It felt like a game; she would pursue and he would run away. The harder she tried, the more he backed off.

Stell was worried and puzzled. She didn't buy into his statement that he was "okay." Normally, he was not a talkative guy, but now he was much quieter than usual at home, and he wasn't sleeping or eating well. Even more confusing was the fact that while he wouldn't talk to her, he would talk freely to other fire fighters. She could hear him on the phone, and that hurt her feelings. She wanted to be the one he confided in.

Communication problems between men and women, especially when it comes to emotions, can be traced back to differences in how we're raised. In the United States boys are trained to hide their feelings. If they don't, they're mocked or labeled "crybabies." The message is clear: it's better to avoid showing your feelings by joking around or pretending they don't exist.

Fire fighters are constantly testing each other's ability to suck up emotions as a way to predict who will stay cool in a stressful situation. Feelings like fear and sadness are associated with doubt and hesitancy. Doubt and hesitancy mean trouble in an emergency. Sometimes emergency responders become so adept at turning off their emotions at work that they find it difficult to turn them back on again when they get home.

Feelings are physical as well as emotional. Men have shorter fuses, meaning it's easier for them to get upset and harder for them to calm down when talking about stressful topics. Women, in contrast, feel better when they ventilate their feelings. By the time we meet and marry, men and women have dissimilar ways of communicating their feelings and different needs in their relationship to one another.

It was a difficult time for Stell. She felt responsible for Rand's well-being and she was certain that talking, just getting things off his chest, would help. She worried that keeping so much emotion inside might set him up for a heart attack or a major depression. But at a certain point she simply gave up and stopped pushing. She told herself that she needed to believe him and trust that his background and training would be sufficient to get him through this crisis. While she never bought into the idea that he wasn't deeply affected by what he saw, she had to accept the fact that he handled his emotions differently than she would under similar circumstances. It seemed enough for him to tell the story over and over without focusing on his feelings.

Rand was invited to make several professional presentations about the crash. Stell went along with him. It helped her to understand what happened and increased her respect for Rand's competency. She always suspected that part of the reason he didn't talk much was to protect her from the gory details of what he had seen. When she attended some of his talks, she realized that he was right: there really were things she didn't want to hear about.

Fire fighters frequently worry about upsetting their families by sharing horrific information. They think it's unfair to burden their loved ones with the consequences of a profession they didn't choose. This is not just kind, it is enlightened self-interest: if your family really knew what you did on the job, they might try to make you quit. Unfortunately, some men don't "get" that what's most important to their wives is a reading on their emotional state rather than a full report about what happened.

Now Stell handles her relationship with Rand in another way. She still pushes him a bit, checks in on him regularly, and observes his behavior. But when he appears to be upset, rather than insisting on talking, she suggests they go to a movie or get to bed early. Instead of hitting the issue straight on, she distracts him with some pleasant, lighthearted activity. This is a perfectly legitimate strategy supported by recent research that indicates that dwelling on problems may be both harmful and ineffective. In fact, psychologists now think the absence of prolonged strong emotions may be a positive sign rather than an indication of denial, callousness, or superhuman self-control. Still, it's sometimes hard for families to know the difference (see Chapters 10 and 11).

HUMOR

Blood and gore all over the floor and me without my spoon.
—ANONYMOUS

I'm hanging around the apparatus bay after dinner. There's a whole lot of joking going on, some of it possibly for my benefit. Most of the humor settles on one fire fighter who is apparently legendary for his huge appetite and his compulsive need to eat on a regular schedule. Everyone, from the chief on down, is ragging on him.

A lot of the kidding is about smells: feet smells, fart smells, and who smells up the bathroom. I ask if anyone ever takes offense at the kidding because it seems pretty brutal at times. I'm told that fire fighters don't let on if they're mad or hurt, because if they did they'd get more of the same. The only truly hurtful thing would be if no one played a joke on you; the accepted norm seems to be that kidding and practical jokes are a sign of affection and a way to release the tension of living and working together.

But sometimes the joking backfires. Kidding around can camouflage truly awful behavior that hurts and humiliates everyone. What's humorous to one person may feel like punishment or harassment to another. Take "butt ball," for example. As a consequence of losing a game of toss, fire fighters in this fire house had to wash dinner dishes with their pants down and a rubber ball encased in a latex glove clenched between their bare cheeks. Anyone who refused to play was banished from eating with his coworkers. What about hazing? Does trying to handcuff and hog-tie a sleeping female fire fighter in the middle of the night constitute harmless hazing?

Is this kind of behavior the exception or the rule? That depends on who you're talking to and where they work. Most fire departments and fire fighters would never tolerate such activities. They insist that fire fighters modify their legendary practical joking and find more respectful and socially acceptable ways to kid around. This change isn't always welcomed, of course. One veteran fire fighter told me that "PCC—that political correctness crap" was wrecking fire fighters' ability to have a good time on the job. "People's sensitivities be damned," he said. "A fire fighter

28

better be agreeable, because if we find his weak spot, he'll get hammered."

Joking is another test of a fire fighter's ability to stay cool, a demonstration that he or she is in control and can be trusted in dangerous situations. The testing is endless. If pranksters run out of imagination or inspiration they can actually purchase a book on firehouse pranks with 122 pages of detailed instructions.

There is an infinite variety of mischief afoot. Fire fighters have a special fondness for aquatic ambush—for example, the unsuspecting fire fighter opens her locker and trips a bucket of water that's been hidden overhead. A fire fighter who's afraid of snakes might find one tied to the steering wheel of his car or coiled inside a soup pot on the night he is scheduled to cook. Fire fighters have found raw eggs in the toes of their boots when they jumped out of bed in the middle of the night. Their turnouts may have been drenched and frozen, their sheets shorted, their clothes thrown out the window, or the slats removed from their beds so that the mattress falls to the floor as soon as they lay down. They put fake "For Sale" signs in front of each other's houses, plant dead fish under the seats of their personal cars, string toilet paper in their buddies' front yards, and start water balloon or food fights.

Families may not understand firehouse humor, which can be blunter and harsher than the kind of humor that goes on at home. Al is well aware of this. When he warned someone in the fire station not to touch the cookies he brought from home for lunch, he knew—as did everyone else—that his warning was tantamount to a direct invitation for the other fire fighters to eat them all. At home, he wouldn't dream of eating someone else's special food.

Families don't sign on for this kind of teasing and they don't need to be tested in the same way fire fighters test each other. John complained a lot that his wife, Anne, was too fat. She dropped by the station one day and the other fire fighters asked her to turn around. "You're not that fat," they told her. She left in tears, feeling humiliated and betrayed. Not surprisingly, she and John had a big fight when he came home.

There's another type of joking that is open to being misunderstood by families: gallows humor. Most emergency responders make puns and jokes about what they see on the job. This is their way of putting emotional distance between themselves and the victims. This kind of humor is best kept in the workplace. It sounds awful to your family to hear burn victims referred to as "crispy critters." And most people would go into shock if they knew that some fire fighters who had just responded to a hanging were back at the firehouse cheerfully singing a country song about a man who hung himself.

Most fire fighters are careful about joking around in public, especially in front of the victim's family, but among themselves gallows humor is a way to blow off tension. Sometimes the best and only thing you can do in the face of an absurd or tragic event is to laugh. There are exceptions: almost any incident involving children or the death of another fire fighter.

Fire fighters encounter a lot of strange things in their careers. They are really astute in finding humor where others can only see pathos and this helps them to bounce back after a nasty encounter.

Humor is also a face-saving way to begin serious conversations and self-disclosures, the kinds of conversations that women often relish and men try to avoid. Phil was sick of eating with the TV blaring. He wanted dinner to be an opportunity to strengthen his all-male crew and bring his guys closer together. He began by asking what he called the "question of the night."

At first, his questions were pure locker-room: "How many times did you crap today?" or "When was the first time you masturbated?" But with time his questions grew more serious: "When was the first time you realized you loved your parents?" There were a variety of reactions to his questions; some guys got teary, others refused to answer. Fire fighters starting calling him on his days off for a question to ask. On the verge of retiring, Phil considers this the biggest achievement of his career and he's proud that younger fire fighters are carrying on the tradition, albeit in a toned-down way that is respectful of a more diversified fire service.

PREOCCUPATION WITH WORK

Some fire fighters are never off duty, which is tough on their families. They live, eat, and sleep fire fighting. This doesn't seem to be a phase, something that will wear off as the novelty of the job wears thin. Sean Flynn, journalist and author, describes this phenomenon in his book *3000 Degrees: The True Story of a Deadly Fire and the Men Who Fought It*:

> Civilians look at a strip mall and see a dry cleaner, a convenience store and a deli . . . firemen see one long box divided into individual compartments connected by a single air space between the roof and the dropped ceilings, a passage for flames to sneak from one shop to the next. Where civilians [see] a hospital, firemen [see] . . . sick people who would need to be carried out. . . . A Wal-Mart or a Home Depot . . . be[comes] a stockpile of flammable synthetics and explosive chemicals stored under a roof held up by . . . a supporting structure that . . . in the heat of a fire could collapse in less than 10 minutes and with little warning." (p. 14)

Kerry says her husband, Grant, a fire fighter/paramedic, thinks about work all the time. When he's home he spends hours surfing the Internet, researching new gadgets and new techniques. He plays on the department softball team and goes to several conventions a year. He listens to the scanner constantly and has been known to leave home to help on a call. He has a reputation as the "neighborhood nurse"; anyone with an injury calls him before they call 911. He talks in codes, using abbreviations and medical terms that Kerry doesn't understand. A kind of mad inventor, he's always building something with or for the other guys on his shift. He wore a pager to their wedding and he wears it when he's lounging around the house in his underwear.

Kerry is philosophical and says fire fighting is not the kind of job you can leave at work. But sometimes she and Grant do fight about his preoccupation with work and the fact that he volunteers for absolutely everything. There are also days when Kerry tells him to get out of her hair and go to the fire station because he's so antsy and preoccupied. She thinks it's nice that he has a place to go. The real rub is that Grant doesn't do as much at home as Kerry does, even though she also works full time and goes to night school. Recently, she took a firm stance and insisted that she needed help. She and Grant engaged in some hard negotiating and they finally agreed that this year he won't play softball for the department when her school starts up again.

GOSSIP: "TELEPHONE, TELEGRAPH, TELL A FIRE FIGHTER"

Fire fighters are proud of being a close-knit group and knowing about each others' moods and private lives. One fire fighter claimed that if a shift-mate was having trouble at home, he'd know about it in less than two hours. On the other hand, there is a lot of complaining about gossip and the need to keep your private life separate or risk having your personal affairs fall into the rumor mill. Tell someone about a fight you had with your wife before work and chances are the other fire fighters won't let it go for years, long after it's been settled. This may make for firehouse fun, but your family may feel differently. In general, fire fighter families don't appreciate having their private lives made "public."

Penny is adamant about this issue based on her own experience. The problem started as a silly domestic quarrel. Penny was mad at her husband, Tony, for leaving her to do the bulk of the housework and demanded he do more. He agreed to help with the laundry. Tony's idea of doing laundry was to throw everything in the washing machine at once. As a consequence he dyed all their underwear pink. It became a private joke that he and Penny wore matching "lingerie" at home. On the spur of the moment, Tony confided this to a fellow fire fighter. Tempted by such a juicy joke, his shift-mate failed to honor the confidence and told everyone in the firehouse.

As a result Penny and Tony, though mostly Tony, were teased about this for years, long after it stopped being funny to them. This was mildly irritating to Tony, but it made Penny wary about trusting anyone at the firehouse with their personal business. She was angry at Tony for his big mouth and she insisted that from then on he keep their personal business to himself. As a result, both their support systems are now smaller than they might have been.

SELF-INFLATION: HEROES AT HOME

Self-inflation is an occupational hazard for most emergency responders. In a closed culture that is constantly reinforcing itself, it is understandable how a fire fighter could confuse doing important *work* with being an important *person*, one whose opinions and needs come before others in the family. Comprehensible? Yes. Acceptable? No.

Jeff told his roommate, Tom, that he considered himself and other fire fighters to be "the gateway between life and death." No doubt he has made a profound difference in victims' lives, but he didn't do it alone, and it certainly didn't give him a pass on behaving with decency and humility at home. And that was the problem: Jeff was acting like a "big man on campus" until Tom told him to get over it. Tom insisted that his job as a teacher was as important and stressful as Jeff's job as a fire fighter, and he said he didn't want to hear Jeff's constant complaints and shoptalk anymore unless he could expect equal airtime. Furthermore, he continued, Jeff's duties at the firehouse didn't relieve him of his obligation to do half of the domestic chores in the apartment they shared.

Self-inflation shows itself in ways besides bragging or expecting others to wait on you. I'm talking to Alice and Jason. They are a strikingly handsome couple: both tall, tanned, and physically fit. They have been married for 10 years and have two children. One, still a baby, is sleeping in his car seat on the floor of my office.

Alice has been struggling with Jason's bossiness. He's a lieutenant at work, and when he's at home he orders everyone around and expects the same compliance he gets at the firehouse. Every decision he makes is a Code 3 (urgent) call: when he tells his wife or their older child to do something, he wants it done right away.

In private, Alice reveals that some of Jason's aggressiveness has rubbed off on her and given her more confidence. She describes herself as timid and passive and says she grew up trying to keep everyone happy. But like many fire fighter spouses, she has toughened up and learned to hold her own. When Jason gets bossy she tells him to "back off." Sometimes when he's in this mood Alice thinks it means he's had a bad day and she tries to get him to talk about it. But if she's had a bad day too it's much harder. On those days, they yell first and talk later.

Jason is controlling in another way. He is admittedly overprotective of his family. He has installed numerous smoke detectors in their home, one every 20 feet, and has placed two fire extinguishers on each floor. His overprotectiveness is most obvious when it comes to their kids. Jason estimates that thus far he has responded to more than 100 incidents involving children who have been raped, shot, beaten, or mutilated. As a result, he watches his children "like a hawk" and never lets strangers talk to them. He knows where they are every minute and with whom. With the help of a cop friend, he illegally obtains background checks on his daughter's teachers and babysitters. He carried out an off-the-cuff inspection of her school. He has a lot of fears—for example, he hates playgrounds because he thinks they are dangerous—he's seen too many children who have fallen and hit their heads—and he worries about stray dogs. On the other hand, sometimes Jason isn't concerned enough. He feels badly about this but he has seen so many gravely injured children that he occasionally finds it hard to sympathize with his daughter when she falls off her bike and scrapes her knee.

Alice appreciates his concerns, but doesn't always share his intensity. She is fearful that he takes things too far and will alienate people or get himself in trouble. When she voices her concerns, sometimes he dismisses her and tells her she's naive and doesn't know what she's talking about. This is both hurtful and inaccurate.

Compared to many fire fighters I know, Jason is a bit overboard with his concerns and the aggressive way he handles them. There is a little bit of Jason in most fire fighters, which is both a blessing and a burden. Being so close to death and injury can make you worry. But it can also fortify your appetite and appreciation for life and clarify your priorities.

Tips for Dealing with Spillover

- Start early on to establish good communication. Learn to assert yourselves, settle disputes, make decisions, and move on before things pile up. Managing a family is like managing an organization. Love isn't enough.
- Talk about talking. Remember: every couple is different and each partner has different needs for communicating. Ask each other:
  - "Are you content with how, when, and where we communicate?"

(continued from previous page)

- "How much detail do we want to share with each other?"
- "Do you want to know when I've been in danger?"
- "Do you want to know when I'm upset?"
- "Do you think we solve problems well?"
- "Do our conflicts get settled satisfactorily?"
- "Is one of us afraid of the other?"
- "Do we each feel listened to?"
- "Do we both have sufficient airtime?"
- "Do our children feel that we listen to them and value their participation in family decisions?"

- If either of you find yourself telling friends and relatives about a problem you're having with your mate before you tell your mate, you're probably not communicating well. It's comforting and helpful to talk with friends and family, but ultimately it won't solve the problem you're having at home. If you're having trouble communicating, consult a therapist (see Chapter 14).

- When listening to each other, resist the temptation to jump in with advice, criticism, or opinions. This is especially hard for professional problem solvers.

- Don't take gallows humor personally, but do assert your rights not to be insulted or drawn into offending others by participating in humor that is racist, sexist, or homophobic— at work or at home. Don't expect your family to embrace pranks like your coworkers—they're not part of that culture. *Never* make family members the object of a joke.

- Set a bottom line about how much shoptalk you can tolerate. Schedule "couple time" when each of you talks about the important issues in your life, but neither of you talks about work.

- Stay in touch with non–fire fighter friends and family, even though scheduling may make this difficult. Avoid becoming isolated. When you have friends outside the department, you can confide in them without worrying about departmental gossip.

(cont.)

(continued from previous page)

- In a crisis, fire fighters probably want to spend more time talking to their coworkers than to their spouses. This can be frustrating and lonely for the spouses. Take care of yourselves and don't focus exclusively on your fire fighters. Think of the safety instructions you get on an airplane: before helping others, first put on your own oxygen mask.
- Don't misjudge a calm, unemotional reaction for callousness or avoidance. Emergency responders have a high tolerance for coping with tragedy.
- Don't accept being told that you don't know what you're talking about because you aren't a fire fighter. They don't know everything either.

CHAPTER 3

Profiles
The Fire Fighter Personality

I walked into Marty's townhouse and knew two things right away: he was a bachelor and he was a fire fighter. His living room was decorated in what might be described as "early fire fighter"; helmets were artfully arranged on one wall and three large framed prints of fire scenes hung over the sofa. His bookshelves were stocked with leather-bound fire-fighting books and fire fighter knickknacks were displayed on every available surface. A woolen blanket with a Dalmatian woven in the center was draped over the arm of an easy chair. His real Dalmatian, Chispa (Spanish for Sparky), bounced around the room, teasing me and the other guests by offering and then retracting her green tennis ball. Photos of Marty dressed in a business suit from his pre-fire-fighting days were relegated to the bathroom.

Fire fighting is not just a job. For many, like Marty, it's a calling and an identity; it defines who he is, on the job and off, both for himself and for his community. On the other hand, there is no such thing as a specific "fire fighter personality." Fire fighters are as different from each other as they are alike. Still, there are a set of attributes or characteristics that many fire fighters share and a set of qualities or features that fire fighters need. Learning about these attributes—the positives and the negatives—may help you understand what motivates fire fighters to seek such challenging work, what they get out of it, and why they sometimes are and sometimes are not easy to live with.

Generally speaking, people who want to be fire fighters are extroverted and friendly. They value teamwork and often love team sports. They have strong needs for companionship and fraternity, which is a good thing because they are joining the "brotherhood," a work family that may, one day, rival their real families. They need strong interpersonal and social skills and the ability to control their anger and tolerate frustration in order to live together and work as a team. From here on out they will be joined at the hip while working, eating, or sleeping.

Certainly, not every fire fighter is social, but even the introverts will have to rise to the occasion when dealing with victims or fellow fire fighters in trouble. Being cooperative is as much a safety issue as it is a social one. Fire fighters who are uncomfortable working with others may hesitate to ask for help during an emergency, exposing themselves to greater risk.

Fire fighters, whether volunteer or career, seem to be physically adept, action-loving risk takers who let their deeds speak for them. They love tools and prefer tinkering with mechanical things to writing reports. This is an advantage because they are dependent upon their equipment to get the job done. They are usually practical, results-oriented, and responsible. They may have high expectations for success and don't suffer failure easily, even in impossible situations. As a result they can be hard on themselves. They are often drawn to the prestige of rescue work, but few are willing to accept public acclaim without a healthy dose of skepticism.

If you asked a dozen people what motivates someone to want to be a fire fighter, you'd probably get a dozen different answers. Many of us would agree that people who want to be fire fighters want to make a difference in the world; but there are some who would say that career fire fighters are vintage blue-collar trade unionists who are equally attracted to the work schedule and the job security. Hardly anyone would suggest people are in it for the money.

FAMILY FOOTSTEPS

What child doesn't look up to fire fighters and admire their shiny equipment? Parents warn misbehaving children that the police will lock them up if they don't straighten out—police really hate to hear parents say this—but they have only good things to say about fire fighters. Fire fighters themselves often radiate contentment and pride to their families, encouraging their children to follow in their footsteps.

Glen Work is a fire chief. He has been taking his son, Tom, to fires since Tom was a toddler. Once when he was a volunteer fire fighter responding to a house fire he left Tom in the car with strict instructions to stay put. He was so involved in putting out the fire that he literally forgot about Tom until the other volunteers began yelling and pointing. He turned around to see Tom, barely six years old and shoeless, standing right behind him, only a few feet from the burning building. Tom is still standing close to his father; today he is a lieutenant in the fire service and they team-teach classes at the fire academy.

Chief Work's own story is different. He became a fire fighter because he was the son of a victim. As a teenager he and four other junior volunteer fire fighters responded to a fire at a supper club. It was a terrible fire: 165 people died in the blaze, including the chief's stepmother. When it was over his grieving stepsister pleaded with him not to ever let anyone else burn to death. Her plea became the basis of his decision to make the fire service his life's work. This is the nature of fire fighters; it is what distinguishes them from the rest of us. They turn *toward* rather than *away from* danger and devastation. Chief Work's personal loss became the impetus for two generations of the Work family to dedicate themselves to fighting fire.

Sometimes the firehouse family fills a gap left by a real family. Jerry's mother died of cancer when he was eight years old, and the firehouse became his second home. Rather than return to an empty house after school, he'd go to the fire station where the fire fighters always had something for him to do and something for him to eat. They were as much fathers to him as his own father, except that they were upbeat and always in a good mood while his father was often depressed and exhausted. Jerry's happiest moments were associated with the fire service. He never considered any other occupation. You can still find Jerry, who has been married and divorced, hanging around the firehouse. He doesn't seem to know what else to do on his days off or where else to take his kids when he has them. One year his shift-mates threw a surprise birthday party for him with a cake and hats and presents. He was a little overwhelmed; it was the first birthday party anyone had ever given him.

COURAGE

I've worked with many police officers. Most officers I know, particularly the young ones, exercise an adaptive state of denial, a mindset that minimizes the risk of death or injury—that is, until someone tries to hurt them or kill them. In contrast, many fire fighters accept, even anticipate, that they are going to be injured on the job. It's one of the reasons, I believe, they're so supportive of each other: they lack the unconscious urge to shy away from an injured or ill colleague in order to preserve their own sense of invulnerability.

Fire fighting attracts people who like to live at the border between order and chaos, who thrive on excitement and exhilaration, who enjoy being in control or restoring control, who gain satisfaction from knowing survival skills. Fire fighting can be a risky business: fire fighters know this from the day they sign on. Having the courage to take risks in the service of helping others is the unspoken contract between fire fighters themselves and between fire fighters and their communities. Taking risks is as much who they are as what they do. It is so natural, so internalized, that fire fighters may have a hard time putting their feelings into words. As a result, families can get a worrisome, lopsided picture: they see the risk, but not the reward.

There's no point in arguing about loving a hazardous job or putting oneself in jeopardy, but there is plenty to be gained from talking and trying to see the whole picture from each other's vantage point. Part of seeing the whole picture is acknowledging that there are many kinds of courage, not all of which involve risk to one's personal safety. Fire fighter families have plenty of courage.

It takes guts to be married to someone who, in times of crisis, may be more available to strangers than to his or her own family. It takes determination to stay home alone at night, fortitude to go to a party by yourself, persistence to be both mother and father, and spunk to say what you really think. It might even take courage for you to read this book.

RISK TAKERS

Around the turn of the century insurance companies issued a metal fire mark to every home they insured. When there was a fire, all freelance fire fighters were paid in proportion to how much of the home they saved. The competition was fierce, because the first engine on scene was the one that got paid. Every fire fighter on duty wanted to be first in the door and they raced each other to the homes that were insured by the best paying companies.

This wasn't just about money. Dangerous work can be exhilarating. People who work in occupations that are exciting as well as hazardous feel good about themselves. They enjoy social prestige and a sense of accomplishment. Families can and should share in this pride. Roofers or foundry workers rarely glory in their perilous work, but it's very common to hear fire fighters exclaim they have the greatest jobs on earth.

On the other hand, some risk takers can invite trouble. Fire fighters who disregard rules, especially safety rules, have more accidents and suffer more injuries. Freelancers who fail to cooperate with their teams are at risk. What is needed is balance. One of my favorite professors in graduate school, Dr. Charles Hampden-Turner, described such balance in terms of an equilibrium between opposites. He said, "Caution without courage is cowardice, and courage without caution is recklessness."

There is a serious downside to the traditional glorification of risk and bravery that some people believe makes the job of fire fighting more dangerous than it has to be. Dr. Burton Clark, training specialist at the National Fire Academy, conducted an opinion survey of 339 academy attendees. He proposed the following scenario: a fire fighter is in a single family detached house wearing self-contained breathing apparatus (SCBA) in an area considered an immediate danger to life and health (IDLH). He then asked, "Under what conditions must this firefighter call 'Mayday'?" ("Mayday" is the universal call of distress. It comes from the French verb *aider*, meaning "to help.")

Ninety-four percent said they would call "Mayday" if they fell through the roof; 92% if they were tangled, pinned, or stuck and couldn't extricate themselves in 60 seconds; 89% if they were caught in a flashover; 88% if they fell through the floor; 82% if they were lost and couldn't see; 69% if their primary exit was blocked or their low air alarm went off and they were 30 seconds from a secondary exit; and 58% if they couldn't find an exit within 60 seconds.

Do you see anything wrong with these answers? What, for instance, is the difference between falling through a roof and falling through a floor in terms of safety? Why wouldn't 100% of the respondents call for help every time? Fire fighters have died or been injured in circumstances just like these. Why take chances?

Dying from Embarrassment

There are many reasons why fire fighters might find it hard to ask for help. Let's start with a basic premise, unproved but widely acknowledged: in a male-dominated culture, asking for help is often considered a sign of weakness.

Ted was working a house fire at 3:00 A.M. He was the company officer. The smoke was very thick and the floor warm. He and his crew crawled down a central hallway and into the basement. Visibility was zero. Ted began to experience trouble with his SCBA gear and thought his oxygen meter was malfunctioning. He panicked, broke out a plywood-covered window, and found himself facing a wall of flame. He was confused and didn't know if he was inside or outside. He had no air and tried to insert his low-pressure hose into his jacket to breathe trapped air, but he couldn't because his fine motor movements had deteriorated due to the lack of oxygen. The next thing he remembers is waking up in an ambulance. Other crew members told him they found him because he was yelling. He was 40 feet from an exit, trying to escape but going the wrong way. When he was interviewed about this incident, he said he didn't ask for help because he was "embarrassed: it was only an ordinary house fire."

There are other reasons, of course, that fire fighters in distress may not call for help. They may be confused, afraid, too focused on their tasks to correctly assess danger, fearful of endangering others, inexperienced, compromised by carbon monoxide or fatigue, or simply in denial. They may also lack the training.

Fire fighters are trained to win, not lose. The message is clear: if you give up, you've failed. The result is that fire fighters have little practice in calling for help, unlike military pilots who routinely practice making tough decisions about ditching their aircraft or ejecting themselves and parachuting to safety.

When Howard fell through the floor into the basement of a burning building, he knew he was required to transmit his location over the radio. He did as instructed. But he radioed "Engine 2 in the basement" in a voice so calm and so controlled that no one realized for quite a while that he had actually fallen into the basement and needed help.

No one is bigger than life, stronger than gravity, or able to defy the laws of physics. It is simply not possible to save every building, put out every fire, or save every victim. On the other hand, believing you can, or believing you should, may be what is required for fire fighters to take risks, get the job done, and bear the heavy historical mantle of courage. This is not something people talk about very often.

A fire service colleague I interviewed thought fire fighters idealized injury and death. Why, he wondered, is there a memorial to fire fighters who died in the line of duty, but no such memorial for dead airline pilots or dead iron workers? "We live up to our risk-taking reputation," he sighed. "There's a reason we are known as the bravest, not the smartest."

I had heard this before. Fire fighters who responded to the Pentagon on 9/11 and suffered no loss of life evidently felt demoralized and overlooked in all the ceremonies honoring the fallen fire fighters of New York City. Taking risks wasn't enough—they felt they had to die to be properly recognized.

LOVE OF TRADITION

Tradition is everything to the fire service. When you understand fire service tradition, you will understand how far the modern fire service has evolved, and how much further it still needs to go. You will understand the magnitude of the changes it faces and why there is often such robust resistance against even the smallest modifications in working conditions.

There are literally hundreds of books about fire service tradition, all tracing a proud history of bravery and promoting the basic fire service values of risk and sacrifice in the service of others—values that are as vital today as they were hundreds of years ago. Almost every fire fighter you meet can tell you the story behind the Maltese Cross, the symbol you see on uniforms and union logos. This special cross is the fire fighter's badge of honor. It means that the fire fighter who wears it is willing to lay down his or her life for someone else.

Traditions fortify us against the unknown and the unexpected. They represent what is predictable and controllable. We are comforted by their sameness because they anchor us in the familiar and the normal. As much as possible families should be included in formal fire service traditions—in fact, honoring the family should be a tradition itself.

The more you are able to participate in fire service traditions like ceremonies and celebrations, the more you will feel connected to your particular department and to the overall fire service mission. It is both a source of pride and resilience to be included in and committed to something larger than yourself.

Including your children in fire service traditions is an opportunity to demonstrate and model social responsibility and commitment to helping others. It is a counterbalance to the self-absorbed materialism promoted by pop culture. Children are inspired by heroes and role models. Those lucky enough to be part of the fire service never face a shortage of either.

Traditions need not be only formal events. Think about developing private family traditions. These can help minimize the disappointment of a missed holiday or special event. They can ease the awkwardness of leave-taking and homecoming. Even a ritual as small as calling home to say goodnight can represent stability and continuity to a child.

HEROICS

Fire fighters claim they don't like being called heroes, that it's embarrassing and undeserved. After all, they're just doing their jobs. "I'm not a hero," one fire fighter insisted, "but I am the last nice guy and the only one to make house calls."

In the aftermath of 9/11, literally every knock on a firehouse door signaled the arrival of grateful citizens bearing cards, banners, and cookies celebrating the bravery and courage of fire fighters everywhere. Fire fighters were touched and appreciative of the attention, although some soon grew weary of it. Others were skeptical of their newfound status. It was as though the public suddenly woke up from a deep sleep and recognized, almost for the first time, the centuries' long contribution of the fire service to public safety.

I asked Eddie, who's been a fire fighter for years, if he thought of himself as a hero and he replied, "Hell, no." He didn't think anyone else did either until 9/11. Just yesterday he was "cussed out" three times by people he went to help. "Nobody wants to pay for you," he said, "until the minute they need you, and then they want you there yesterday." He complained that garbage collectors in his part of the country make more money than he does. Eddie's wife said people have told her they think fire fighters are cold, callous, and abrasive. She thinks the public confuses how fire fighters act in an emergency with their true natures and knows it's an added stress on Eddie to try and live up to the public's sometimes unreal expectations.

In many ways she's right. When fire fighters believe their own press notices they become imprisoned by public perceptions and can pressure themselves to fill the shoes they say they don't want to wear. Sometimes it falls to the family to remind a fire fighter that he is only human or that she is doing the best she can under difficult circumstances. Fire fighters can be tough on themselves. It is truly helpful to know that no matter how others see you or how you see yourself, your family will stick with you, listen to your troubles, and give you feedback you can trust.

HEARTFELT HELPERS

If you're looking for love, join the fire department.
—JOSEPH WAMBAUGH (1992),
author and retired Los Angeles police officer

Early in his career, Curtis was a fire fighter/paramedic. One of his first calls involved a young man in full cardiac arrest. Curtis and his crew tried their best, as they always did, but they couldn't revive the victim, who was probably dead when they arrived. Back at the fire station, Sam, a veteran fire fighter/paramedic, noticed that Curtis was moping around, and was not his usual jovial self. He took Curtis aside and asked him what was wrong. Curtis explained that he was feeling down because he felt like he hadn't done his job. His job, as he saw it, was to save people—anything less was a failure and he didn't easily tolerate failure. This is a common mindset for firefighters. After all, when they "lose," someone else has lost a lot more. Sam was one of those prickly-on-the-outside, soft-on-the-inside type of guys, outspoken and sensitive at the same time. "Get used to it, kiddo," he admonished. "Losing people happens all the time. If you want a long shelf life in this business, you'd better learn that we win some and we lose some. That's the way it is."

Fire fighters want to be of help, and like those in other helping professions—psychologists, for example—they feel best when they are needed and can make a difference. One fire captain told me that he had fought fires in million-dollar homes, but his proudest moment was preserving the belongings of a fire victim who was so poor that he kept all his earthly possessions in one box.

Luke was in my office, eaten up with frustration because his captain had refused to let him trade shifts with another fire fighter so he could take care of some important personal business. This wasn't the first time Luke had come to see me boiling at what he considered a heartless bureaucracy. Sometimes he gave me the impression that he believed he was the only caring person in his department. Since there was no way he could continue to be a fire fighter without working in a bureaucracy, I asked him to tell me what gave him satisfaction about his work. By way of answer, he told me the following story.

He was driving home after work when he came across a family who had run off a busy freeway after their tire blew out. No one was seriously hurt and there was only minor damage to their camper. But Luke stopped to help, checked everyone out, put traffic cones in the road to protect their vehicle, and then drove the family to the nearest gas station. He was happy to help, but when the family wanted to write a letter of appreciation to his department, he refused to allow it. It was quite clear that he got a great deal of gratification from helping and was proud of himself, proud that he took the time and proud that he had the ability to make a difference. All he's ever wanted to do, he told me, ever since he was a child, was to make a difference in someone's life. As he said this he had tears in his eyes.

Fire fighters want to be needed and they like to be liked, just like the rest of us. Dan's lifelong goal was to be a cop. He studied criminology in college and spent several years working as a sheriff's deputy. When he and his wife moved closer to her parents, there were no police jobs in the area, so Dan reluctantly hired on at the local fire department thinking it would be a stepping-stone back to a law enforcement job. The day he started, his attitude changed. Suddenly he had a job where people loved him even when he broke their windows, smashed their furniture, got water all over their belongings, and blew diesel exhaust in their faces. It was like heaven compared to law enforcement where, if he did his job right, everyone was angry at him or at each other. Even the people he helped when he was a deputy associated him with something terrible. One time, in a restaurant, he ran into a woman whose child had been kidnapped. He had spent hours talking with her and felt very sympathetic about her ordeal. He said hello in the restaurant and as soon as she realized who he was, she burst into tears and ran into the rest room. He felt terrible for upsetting her.

Compared to cops, who have a mandate to control people and put bad guys in jail, fire fighters enjoy much more positive interactions with the public. There are exceptions, of course; some people may not be pleased to see arson investigators and fire marshals, the enforcement arm of the fire service. Fire fighters and emergency medical services (EMS) personnel have been abused, assaulted, or even murdered in the line of duty by the very people they have come to help. But, in general, people are happy to see fire fighters coming. Fire fighters do best when they are comfortable being in a positive limelight.

Wendell is a great example. We are on our way to a preschool. Wendell has been asked to make a safety presentation as part of his public education duties. He welcomes the opportunity because he truly believes that making a positive impression on young children ensures their future safety and helps with recruiting and community relations as well. He has gifts to distribute: badges, plastic helmets, balloons, and coloring books that he hopes will serve as a reminder of today's lesson: never play with matches. Wendell doesn't have any kids of his own, but he handles the group easily as he teaches them to "stop, drop, and roll" if there's a fire. In this miniaturized environment, Wendell is bigger than life, the center of attention for two dozen enrapt children and their teachers.

Wendell handles a lot of his department's community programs, like public education and media relations. He is very good at what he does and very much at ease in the spotlight. In our official vehicle, on the way to and from the preschool, he honks and waves at people on the street and in passing cars. They all wave back. We stop for lunch at a local restaurant, where he is a celebrity. The waitresses all know him and a half-dozen customers stop by our table to say hello. He is beaming and doesn't seem to mind that his food is getting cold. I ask him if he sometimes wishes he could eat his lunch in peace. "Never," he says. "This is what it's all about."

CHAPTER 4

Climbing the Career Ladder

From Recruitment to Retirement

The young boy looked up at the fire fighter and said, "When I get to be a grownup, I want to be a fireman like you."

"I'm sorry, son," the fireman replied, "but you can't be both."
—quoted in MAYNARD GOOD STODDARD,
"The Art of the Fire Fighter"

It's morning break time and there are several fire fighters sitting around the coffee table reading newspapers. The guys are young except for Chad, who is nearly 60 years old and looks it. Fire fighting has been hard on his body. Someone asks Chad when he's going to retire and he replies, "Not any time soon—I'm still having fun." Chad is not unusual; many fire fighters love their jobs for their entire careers. The job of fire fighting seems to sustain people rather than deplete them. There are volunteer fire fighters who are still at it in their seventies and eighties.

Fire fighters' careers evolve in topsy-turvy ways; stress is highest in the beginning when fire fighters are at their physical peak. By the time they have the wisdom, skill, and confidence to be really good at their jobs, their bodies are starting to wear down. Unlike other careers where people strive to get promoted and are devastated when they fail, with some exceptions, line-level fire fighters actually seem happier than those who do make the move from blue shirt to white.

Whatever career choices fire fighters make affects their families, and therefore should be selected with everyone's input. Fire fighters and their families can make better decisions when they know the territory and can anticipate the inevitable challenges of a long career.

This chapter lays out the various stages of a fire fighter's career. Bear in mind, however, that this is a map, not a timetable. Everyone will chart his or her own course differently. A lot of what happens in a fire fighter's career depends on many things:

- The job itself—meaning its physical, social, and emotional demands
- The call volume and the type of calls
- The amount of control a fire fighter can exert over these demands
- The organizational culture and leadership style of his or her organization
- The relationship between the department and the community it serves
- Individual factors such as personality, coping style, stress management skills, available support systems, health, and financial stability
- And last, but not least, *luck!*

FIRST RUNG: GETTING THE JOB

The hardest part of being a paid fire fighter may be getting the job in the first place. Fire fighting is a coveted job. There are 500–1,000 applicants for every open position. In some places it's many times harder to get into the fire academy than it is to get into an Ivy League college. By contrast, the volunteer fire service is perpetually looking for applicants and the screening process is comparatively simple and welcoming; applicants are voted in or appointed by incumbent volunteers or staff. Because volunteerism is on the decline, few people are turned away.

Getting a professional fire-fighting job is a competitive and stressful process. Candidates face a series of daunting challenges that their predecessors never had to confront. By the time applicants successfully pass all the requirements, they are deservedly proud of themselves. They have reached the first rung of a ladder to membership in an elite group.

The first hurdle is getting an application form. Tommy camped out in front of city hall for two days and two nights just to be sure he'd get one. Fire-fighting jobs were so popular that the department he wanted to join purposely limited the number of application forms it distributed in order to avoid being overwhelmed by job seekers. Once he had the coveted documents in hand, he spent weeks filling them out and gathering proof that he met the entry-level requirements. His girlfriend, Candace, a college student, helped him when she could.

After his application was accepted, Tommy had to submit to a background investigation of his personal and professional history in order to prove he was a person of integrity and character. The interview was a "mind twister"; the investigator asked him all sorts of odd and intrusive questions about his sexual activities. Tommy was only 22 years old, and he had led a fairly sheltered life guided by religious principles. The whole thing was embarrassing and sometimes he didn't even understand the questions. When he told Candace about it, she found the questions offensive.

Because he was a college graduate, Tommy had no trouble passing the next step: a written test that covered basic math, English, mechanical reasoning, physics, and general knowledge. The physical agility test was more of a challenge. While it was a fair test developed by incumbent fire fighters, Tommy heard it favored applicants with previous fire-fighting experience, athletic training, or experience in jobs involving similar physical activity. So he spent months working out, building cardiovascular endurance and muscle strength. He joined others for practice sessions at the fire department gym where a mentor was helping eager applicants prepare for the test. He and Candace saw each other less and less.

The Candidate Physical Agility Test

The department Tommy wanted to join used the Candidate Physical Ability Test (CPAT). The CPAT is a grueling, standardized, continuous sequence of events that simulates critical fire-fighting tasks. The test was developed in 1996 as part of the Joint Labor

Management Wellness and Fitness Initiative sponsored by the International Association of Firefighters (IAFF) and the International Association of Fire Chiefs (IAFC). Its objective is to identify trainable candidates who are physically able to perform essential job tasks at fire scenes. It is so strenuous that applicants are required to sign a release and a waiver form to take the CPAT and another one to go home afterward.

In order to pass, applicants must complete eight tasks within 10 minutes and 20 seconds while wearing a 50-pound vest that simulates the weight of SCBA breathing equipment and firefighter protective clothing. Twenty seconds are allotted between tasks for rest and recovery. The eight tasks are as follows (for a more complete description, see Resources).

1. Stair climb (wearing an additional 25-pound hose pack)
2. Ladder raise
3. Hose drag
4. Equipment carry
5. Forcible entry
6. Victim search
7. Rescue drag
8. Ceiling pull

Tommy passed the CPAT with flying colors. He and Candace went out to celebrate. She was happy for him, but he was delirious and the whole evening had a sort of lopsided feeling to it. Candace confessed that she was tired of hearing about the fire department. She felt as though her stress and her studies were not as important as what Tommy was going through. She wasn't sure she could stay the course.

Tommy had accomplished a lot, but he was still far from finished. At this point, the names of all eligible candidates were placed on a rank-ordered, time-limited list. As openings occurred, candidates from the top of the list would be interviewed by the fire chief and a panel of fire fighters, given a conditional job offer, and then required to take medical and psychological examinations. It seemed to Tommy and Candace that this process was taking forever. Candace especially resented not being able to make plans. Tommy reassured her that his process was actually moving faster than he expected. In some departments it could take years! He told her about a friend of his who was on a list for so long it expired before his friend was ever called for an interview. Candace was not comforted by this news.

Tommy pressed on. He studied in preparation for his interviews. When he was finally called in he found the fire fighter panel to be a cinch, but the chief's interview threw him for a loop. He had expected to be asked all sorts of technical questions about fire suppression and building construction. Instead the chief wanted to know about Tommy's personal life, his family, and his education. The interview ended and Tommy couldn't tell if he'd passed or failed. When the letter with a conditional offer of employment arrived, he was so elated that he wasn't even nervous about making an appointment for psychological screening.

Psychological Testing

For the past 40 years police officers have been screened for character, integrity, and intelligence. They have been subjected to a whole array of invasive investigative procedures such as polygraphs, urine testing, psychological interviews, and so on. By contrast, fire fighters have only recently been evaluated for qualities beyond physical strength and basic intelligence. The most notable addition—implemented primarily in large urban departments—is the psychological assessment of stability and suitability.

Psychological testing has met with a lot of resistance. It is the final hurdle in the hiring process and creates a lot of anxiety and resentment. The personnel director of a large urban department recently told a colleague of mine that when police officer candidates fail their psychological evaluations, they're ashamed to admit it to their peers. But when fire fighters fail their "psychs," they broadcast it to everyone they know as proof that the psychologist who tested them is nuts. And then, he added, they go on to sue everybody involved.

Several major changes in the fire service have prompted the use of preemployment psychological screening. Two of the most prominent developments are the inclusion of women and minorities and the incorporation of emergency medical services into the fire service. Just because applicants are strong enough and smart enough to do the job doesn't mean that they will be able to change with the times, live and work well with people different from themselves, or cope with the high stress associated with providing emergency medical care (see Chapter 5).

Fire fighting, like policing, has become more community-oriented and geared toward customer service. Fire prevention efforts have been so successful that modern fire departments must expand their services in order to justify the expense of keeping a well-equipped fire force waiting for a fire emergency. Fire suppression may be an applicant's major interest, but his or her future employer wants to know that the applicant has a wide range of interpersonal skills and can interact with the public in a variety of ways, all of which will reflect on the department. In these days of fiscal crises, almost all government agencies have to be creative in order to recover some of their costs. Volunteer departments have always faced this challenge.

The events of 9/11 and growing concerns over homeland security have only intensified the need for fire fighters to have solid interpersonal skills. The potential for future terrorist attacks has forced cooperation and planning between independent public safety disciplines that have historically not worked together often or well. Traditional turf battles are unacceptable where public safety is concerned. What is required is sophisticated communication, collaboration, and organizational skills.

Because it is a relatively new science, psychological screening is probably better at screening out problem applicants than predicting who will be a good fire fighter.

There are a number of essential characteristics and abilities that psychologists look for in potential fire fighters. I've summarized them so you can see just how far the role of fire fighter has evolved. Volunteer fire fighters are not required to undergo this kind of screening, but they may still be held to these same standards.

1. Understand, remember, and implement complex instructions in normal and crisis situations.
2. Maintain regular attendance and be punctual.
3. Work independently.
4. Exercise good judgment in both normal and emergency situations.

5. Interact and communicate appropriately and effectively with the public, supervisors, and coworkers.
6. Share living and working quarters.
7. Follow orders explicitly and accept constructive criticism appropriately.
8. Withstand the stress and pressure of life-endangering circumstances on the fireground.
9. Make decisions and maintain composure under highly stressful, frightening, or otherwise upsetting circumstances.
10. Take calculated, but not unnecessary, risks.
11. Be free of abnormal fears (e.g., fear of heights, enclosed spaces) or compulsions (e.g., fire setting).
12. Accept danger and put the safety of citizens above the safety of self.
13. Be aware of hazards and take precautions.
14. Make life-and-death decisions involving self and others.
15. Maintain abstinence from mood-altering chemicals (non-prescribed, controlled, or illegal) while at work.
16. Be free from chemical abuse or dependency.
17. Effectively coordinate sensory experiences and motor activity.
18. Show positive customer service attitudes toward citizens, including being supportive and comforting in times of stress or crisis.
19. Exercise honesty and integrity in all interactions with the public, peers, and supervisors.
20. Work within a paramilitary command structure; accept authority and obey orders without undue friction or resentment.
21. Conscientiously perform routine, even boring, tasks and duties.
22. Within reason, work in spite of fatigue and pain.
23. Maintain a high standard of ethical personal conduct.

There are a few things missing from this list, items that are obviously important but not easily mandated: dedication to the job, support from family and friends, flexibility, a life outside the job, a philosophical or spiritual life, and a sense of humor.

Tommy easily passed his medical and psychological exams.

He felt like the "King of the World." He had wanted to be a fire fighter as far back as he could remember and now he was finally on his way. Candace was happy and hopeful. The long wait was over, Tommy had what he wanted, and she expected to have what she wanted too: more of his time and attention.

SECOND RUNG: LEARNING THE ROPES

"Can't make me quit, ain't no way, like stink on a monkey, I'm here to stay."
— RECRUIT CHANT, Tucson Fire Department

Tommy remembers his academy training as 20 weeks of the "best stress I ever had." He was living his dream. Still on study mode from college, he sailed through the classes on fire science, building construction, radio communications, standard operating procedures, arson investigation, fire inspection, public education, computers, report writing, emergency vehicle operations, and basic emergency medical science such as anatomy, physiology, pathology, and pharmacology.

The learning curve was steep and he enthusiastically soaked up everything. Doing well was the most important thing in his world and he gave it 150% of his time and energy. Candace literally dropped off his radar screen. The few times they saw each other Tommy would go over to her apartment, eat dinner, and immediately fall asleep on her couch. They never went out, they never saw friends, they never made love.

Candace felt betrayed; they had been dating for six years, but now Tommy seemed to feel closer to his academy mates than he did to her. He certainly spent more time with them, studying and talking each other through the rough spots. When Candace needed him, he wasn't there for her, physically or emotionally. When she wanted to talk, he seemed resentful and gave her the feeling that she was taking him away from more important things. She stopped calling as often and began making weekend plans with other friends.

At the academy Tommy was being socialized into the fire service—meaning that he had to show everyone that he could and would try with all his heart and never give up. Some days it was almost unbearable to be dressed in full turnouts drilling in the hot sun for hours, pulling hose line from the truck, hoisting it on his shoulder, laying it down in neat lines, dragging it up stairs, or hooking it to a hydrant. And then when it was charged—filled with hundreds of gallons of pressurized water and bucking like a horse—he had to aim it at a selected target. It was like wrestling with the wind; even small lines can break a fire fighter's arm or leg.

The endless drilling strained as well as strengthened everybody. Each drill had potential for a disabling injury that could mean the end of someone's career. Some days the class had to crawl through live fire burns where temperatures ranged to 1,000 degrees and the superheated air created lethal steam. It was a simulation, but it was terrifyingly real.

Blindfolded, Tommy and his classmates practiced rescuing themselves, each other, and victims. They studied techniques for an endless variety of complex situations: confined-space fires, gas fires, high-rise fires, hazardous material spills, wildland fires, and fires where there is no available water. They raised, lowered, and carried heavy ladders back and forth, up and down. And when they were finished, they did it again. They practiced search-and-rescue techniques in all kinds of diabolical scenarios. They mastered automobile extrication and learned to use powerful tools to remove people trapped in crushed cars—all without killing the victims or getting themselves knocked flat by exploding air bags.

As the weeks went on, the pressure increased. Every skill test or written exam was a challenge. One failure could lead to automatic dismissal. Two of Tommy's classmates dropped out; another wrenched his knee so badly he needed surgery; a fourth was terminated for cheating on a test.

And then it was over. The graduation ceremony was impressive and emotional. Tommy's whole family was there. So was Candace. The chief made a moving speech. He told the audience that there is no more honorable profession than fire fighting, that it is the best job in the world. He said that in a sad and cynical world fire fighters are still regarded as heroes because the work they have chosen is about risking their lives in order to save others. He promised that they could and would make a difference in the world. He paid scant attention to what their families might have to sacrifice in the process.

There were cookies and punch. Families milled around the academy and toured the facilities. The new fire fighters—they were no longer called "recruits"—discussed their future assignments. After all this time together they would be going to different departments or different shifts. There was a party scheduled later that night, a time to cut loose and celebrate. Tommy had forgotten to tell Candace about it until graduation. When he asked her to go, she told him that she had made other plans. It was clear that their relationship was over. They had both gotten a preview of how much this job demands and an opportunity to try the fire service lifestyle on for size. Tommy loved it, Candace did not. They were sad, but relieved to have found this out before getting married.

Most of Tommy's fellow graduates had a different experience. Their mates were thrilled that they were closer to an exciting job that had status and security. They were optimistic about the future: if there were downsides to this life, they were outweighed by the benefits. Tommy hoped that one day he'd find someone who appreciated the fire fighter lifestyle and he vowed to do a better job tending to their relationship.

THIRD RUNG: PROBATION

> Well, first they got to take the test. And then there's this
> brutalizing physical. And paperwork, lots of paperwork.
> Piles of paperwork. And then they go home and wait.
> Long, long wait. They think it'll never end. Most of the
> guys get rejected. But if you're lucky, you get the call. . . .
> Come on down. You're in. . . . And then you start. You sit
> down, keep your eyes open and shut up.
> —NICK, in *The Guys*

Probationary fire fighters, paid and volunteer, are like bugs under glass. The eyeballing is mutual. The veteran fire fighters are trying to show the "probies" what it means to be a good fire fighter in that particular house, on that particular shift, in that particular department. At the same time, the probies are trying to convince the veterans and themselves that they measure up and are fit to work and live with. It's hazardous territory; one mistake can ruin your reputation and earn you a "jacket" (a bad name or negative notoriety) you won't easily lose.

Firehouse Etiquette

There are certain conventions demanded in the fire service, and the sooner probies catch on, the better. It was only Hal's third shift and he'd already offended four people. His initial mistake was to call the captain by his first name, presuming a familiarity he hadn't earned. The irate captain told him, "You don't get to join the club until you've nailed some boards on the clubhouse wall." As if that wasn't bad enough, Hal sat in a senior fire fighter's favorite recliner without asking permission and read the newspaper when the dishwasher needed to be emptied. In no time he'd earned a jacket as a typical Gen X slacker.

A veteran fire fighter took Hal aside and sat him down for a lesson in firehouse etiquette. When it was over, Hal had a long list of instructions to follow: "Don't take the job for granted. Don't kid around until you've earned our respect. Be on time—shaved, showered, and ready to work. Don't watch TV, talk on the phone, surf the net, or work out before 4:00 P.M. Don't fart in the rigs. Before you sit down, ask whose chair this is. Before you choose a bed, check to see which bed is available. Keep your tools clean. Pick up after yourself. Hang up your turnouts when you're done and never borrow anyone's equipment. Don't talk shit about other fire fighters. Replace things you use up, like toilet paper. On your birthday cook dinner for everyone. When you pull an over-time shift, buy dessert. Start doing housework without being asked and don't expect anyone to help you, especially when cleaning the bathrooms. Offer to cook. Pay your house-fund dues on time. When you get up, raise the flag, empty the dishwasher, make coffee, and put the newspapers on the table. Never criticize a senior fire fighter, even if you know more than he does, and never let a senior fire fighter beat you to a ringing telephone."

It was a tough lesson, but it gave Hal the guidance he needed to turn things around. He went from being friendly to being respectful. To his shift-mates this was a sign that he was willing to take orders and be part of a team—it was a minor change but it spoke volumes about who he was and how he could be counted on. He started getting up at 4:00 A.M. so he could make coffee for his captain, who was an early riser. By the time his probation was over he went from being known as the "slacker" to being called the "sprinter" because he would race to be first to answer the telephone.

Over the years, Hal and his family will reap benefits from his learned generosity and willingness to pitch in. Working hard and helping others virtually ensures that your fellow fire fighters will be there when you need them to help put a new roof on your house or tile your bathroom. They'll be there to hold a golf tournament to raise money for your sick child, landscape your backyard when you're laid up, look after your family when you die, or cover for you when your back hurts and you don't want the boss to know just how bad it really is.

First Fire

In the beginning, they all want to be heroes. Even before they enter their first fire, they will have secretly placed their helmets in the ovens at home to soften them up a bit—to dull and char and melt them, slightly, so anxious are they for combat and its validations; its contract with their spirit. Kirby remembered the first house fire . . . his new shiny suit yellow and clean amongst the work-darkened suits of the veterans. . . . After that fire he drove out into the country and set a little grass fire, a little piss-ant one that was in no danger of spreading, then put on his bunker gear and spent all afternoon walking around in it, dirtying his suit to just the right color of anonymity.

—RICK BASS, "Fireman"

It was six months before Jenna caught her first real fire and it was a big one, a house fire in a heavily wooded and hilly section of the county. Her department had been going door to door serving notice to the residents that it was their responsibility to clear debris away from their property lines, remove underbrush, trim back trees, and keep the dried grasses mowed. Some of the newer houses had sprinkler systems, but there were older homes, cabins really, that were tinderboxes.

A tortuous trip edging slowly up the narrow winding roads

gave Jenna a lot of time to work up anxiety. She knew everyone was going to be watching her to see how fiercely she fought the fire.

Veterans in her company were skeptical about women serving in the fire service. While they were superficially friendly, she was going to have to prove herself to them physically, on the fireground. Her plan was to get the coveted position of being first in, and that meant she'd have to jump off the truck and grab the nozzle. It was not her nature to be that aggressive—the guys in her academy class were always elbowing each other out of the way and showing off for their instructors—but her mentor, Ron, had warned her. "Everyone's going to be waiting to see you bust your cherry on a fire, so you'd better be ready cause you won't get a second chance." Jenna had winced at the crude allusion to losing her virginity, but she liked Ron and trusted him.

By the time they pulled up, the empty house was fully engaged, with black smoke everywhere. Jenna leaped from the truck, mask and gear in place, and as soon as the company officer yelled for a line she grabbed the nozzle and started forward. It was hotter than hell and pitch-black inside. The house was like a maze, overfilled with furniture. Jenna dropped to her knees and started crawling around and over whatever was in her path. She was sucking up air at a rapid rate. Something crashed to her right. She could hear people yelling at her but couldn't make out exactly what they were saying. She'd never been so scared. It was tempting to start blasting water to cool things down, but she didn't want to create steam or waste water until she found the seat of the fire.

The fire went to five alarms, mutual aid arrived from four adjoining departments, the electrical company showed up, and so did the police, the chaplain, people from the department of forestry, and someone from animal control. The house and all its contents were a total loss, but fire fighters kept the woods from catching fire and saved the neighbor's new garage and in-law unit. Someone made a joke about fire fighters being foundation savers. Several fire fighters congratulated Jenna for doing a good job.

This was not like any drill Jenna had ever been in. Drills have beginnings and endings, but this operation went on for five hours, mostly devoted to overhauling (tearing down) the smoking, sopping-wet roof and peeling back the charred walls looking for hidden hot spots that might reignite. Jenna had never been so tired. She kept waiting, in vain, for her adrenaline to kick in and give her a second wind. Several times she thought she might throw up or collapse, but she never did. That night, back at the firehouse, Jenna celebrated her first big fire in the traditional way by buying dessert for everyone in the house. Her selection? A cherry pie.

FOURTH RUNG: THE EARLY YEARS

Probation was over and Zach finally had tenure. The job was securely his and he wasn't being constantly scrutinized or tested. Life was suddenly so easy it felt wrong. Work wasn't just easy, it was exhilarating. Zach lived for fires and emergencies. Every ringdown (alarm) was a novel experience and a chance to learn something new. He talked shop endlessly with his shift-mates. He felt so totally fulfilled that he could imagine himself happily doing this forever. He had a few "saves," which were intoxicating and left him with a sense of power over people's lives. In contrast, his off days were a real letdown. He was bored and didn't know what to do with himself now that he wasn't studying every minute. He listened to the scanner constantly and found excuses to drop by the fire station.

These early years are filled with excitement and a growing sense of self-confidence. It is a time when new fire fighters, whether career or volunteer, build and strengthen their skills, figure out how to balance home with work, come to understand the rewards and responsibilities of saving lives, and learn how and when to take charge of a situation. It is a time when some families may feel like they are taking a backseat to the fire service and that their lives pale in comparison with work.

There were numerous incidents that first year when Zach was forced to take charge. Family members were the worst for interfering and being hysterical. Even good samaritans sometimes made trouble: on one occasion a doctor stopped to assist at a freeway wreck and Zach wound up ordering him to leave the scene because he was interfering with standard protocols. An angry crowd at a multiple-fatality fire had to be forcefully moved to allow equipment through, at which time they began pelting the fire fighters and cops with bottles and rocks. Drunks were frequently combative and resisted treatment, especially the "regulars" who were always falling or getting into fights.

Fire fighters at this stage have to take care that they are not confident to the point of being arrogant or overbearing. Zach imagined that other people listened to him with more respect. Sometimes he had a mental image of himself as a superman, ax in hand. He was embarrassed by these feelings, but when he told his minister, his minister kindly and wisely suggested that the hero image was a symbol for the genuine pleasure Zach experienced knowing that he was trained and able to restore control when control was lost.

Zach is a fire fighter/paramedic. One day, after dropping off a patient in the ER, Zach met Lynda, an intensive care nurse. They began dating. After six months they moved in together. Zach had been a committed bachelor and had never lived with anyone before. He found it hard to switch gears between work and home. Wherever he went everyone loved and respected him. Going home could be a "downer," especially after an exhilarating day. Sometimes he found it difficult to settle in long enough to sort laundry and walk the dog. There were a lot of days when he grew bored with ordinary conversation and frankly missed being the center of attention. He felt as if he was living off admiration and adrenaline.

From Lynda's point of view, fire fighter/paramedics were out of touch with reality. Their job is to swoop in, load, and go—put the patient on a gurney and make a mad dash for the ER—and not hang around long enough to see the ultimate results. She told Zach that the real heroes were nurses like herself who provided bedside care and comfort to frightened, desperately ill patients and their families, day after discouraging day. Zach had an urge to fight back, but he had seen some of Lynda's patients when he visited her floor and truthfully he couldn't imagine himself having the patience or compassion Lynda had.

Zach was struggling to find balance in his life. His firehouse had a "club atmosphere" and things sometimes deteriorated to the "lowest common moral denominator." There was a lot of bar hopping and partying. Being a fire fighter seemed to have made him a magnet for women. At first that was a bonus, but now it was making trouble. Zach felt torn between being with the guys and building a life with Lynda. He wondered if he was starting to drink too much and too often. Some of his friends had affairs and were divorced.

Zach made a tough decision: at the first opportunity he moved to a different firehouse. The atmosphere in his new house was quieter and his shift-mates were more family-oriented, interested in building stable family lives and solid futures. There was less talk about women and more talk about financial investments and real estate. Zach didn't feel as torn between going home or staying out with the guys. He grew confident in his ability to settle down and have children. He proposed to Lynda on her birthday and they got married on his.

FIFTH RUNG: THE MIDDLE YEARS

The middle years are a quiet time for most, but not all, fire fighters. Things get easier and more comfortable. Experience begins paying off. Fire fighters at this stage know what they are doing on the job. They don't have to put a lot of thought and energy into work and can redirect their energies to their families.

After Herb and Lorraine had their first child, Herb was as engrossed with the baby as he ever was with fire fighting. His days off were devoted to his daughter. As a younger fire fighter he wanted to experience everything and he was vexed during slow periods when there were too few fires to fight and too few medical calls. Now he appreciated the slow periods and the opportunity to relax. The only bad part was that calls involving dead or injured children seemed a hundred times worse since he had a child of his own.

At the same time—and this is a common paradox—he began to worry that he was growing "stale." He told Lorraine that he lacked the compassion he used to feel for victims and their families. Unless it was a child, death didn't shake him up the way it used to. He worried too that he was becoming less sensitive to people in his private life. Only last weekend he had brusquely warned a neighbor's child not to get hurt because he wasn't going to play neighborhood nurse and give medical aid on his days off.

Herb thought back to his experiences as a probie and remembered how shocked he was when a police officer on scene told jokes about necrophilia right in front of a dead body. The other day Herb had responded to the scene of a high-speed car crash. There were badly injured victims trapped in the car and one lying dead on the road. Herb stepped over the dead body to get to the car and heard someone behind him say, "Boy, I hope I never get that cold." The remark hit home; all the rest of that day Herb worried that he was becoming calloused and hard.

When Herb came home the next morning he asked Lorraine if she'd seen a change in him. What she said in response was a surprise. She didn't think he'd become callous—maybe he was slightly more detached, something she expected came with age and experience—but she did think he was bored. Herb was amazed. He loved his job and had been enthusiastic since he was a rookie. "Well," said Lorraine, "maybe you have to be on fire to burn out."

Lorraine was able to give Herb honest and caring feedback based on her intimate knowledge of him as a total person, not just as a fire fighter. This is one way members of families show their support for each other. As a result of this conversation, Herb made an appointment with an employee assistance counselor who suggested that at this point in his career he might need some variety in his work. He encouraged Herb to think about putting in for a promotion.

It was a tough decision. Things were pretty mellow and easy the way they were. Going for a promotion was risky. On the one hand, setting himself a new challenge would be a shot in the arm. On the other hand, if he failed he would have sacrificed countless hours away from his family studying.

Most of Herb's fellow fire fighters seemed content to work as fire fighters and keep themselves occupied off shift with second jobs or hobbies. But he saw what could happen to fire fighters who were afraid to try for promotion or who tried and failed. Some of them grew bitter and stuck. Worse still, they made life hell for the younger supervisors who surpassed them. It was a real morale buster. That was the last thing Herb wanted.

Herb knew there would be dues to pay for climbing the ladder, but he liked learning new things. Once he committed to the idea, he told Lorraine he felt like he was renewing his marriage vows; studying made him feel more involved with work than he had in quite some time. His diligence paid off. There were a number of openings due to retirements and he had no trouble earning promotion to engineer.

By now Herb had more than a decade on the job. At this stage, most fire fighters have settled in, grown up, and calmed down. Many have lost parents and gained children. They are beginning to feel their age in comparison with younger fire fighters. They have a more realistic sense of themselves and profound feelings of responsibility to their families. Their security needs are deeper and broader. They see people in the private sector being laid off during tough economic times and take comfort in the fact that while fire departments are not immune to financial cutbacks, it's rare for senior fire fighters to lose their jobs.

As an engineer, Herb loved the firehouse he was in and the shift he was on. It was very companionable and made coming to work a joy. His schedule allowed him to help out at his children's school. He started a small landscaping business with another fire fighter to supplement his income so that Lorraine could work part time. Like most fire fighters, he enjoyed being busy and being of service, so when the volunteer fire department in his rural community put out a call for volunteers, he joined up. At this point, he and Lorraine decided that their life was in good balance. If he continued to seek and gain promotions, he would eventually move to a 40-hour week and sacrifice time with his children during a long rush-hour commute. They both agreed that moving further up didn't seem worth the money or the effort.

SIXTH RUNG: FROM BLUE SHIRT TO WHITE SHIRT

... There is just about as much stress behind the desk as there is on the end of a nozzle, and it is not nearly as much fun.
—RONNY J. COLMAN, *Going for Gold*

In our culture, upward mobility, accumulation, prestige, and status are ways in which we judge our successes and measure our self-worth. Men, especially, have been saddled with this judgment.

It's very important to make decisions about promotion carefully and with due consideration for your family, your temperament, and the realities of what you're getting into, rather than blindly following some presumed predetermined path.

Rob had been with his department for 12 years. He'd complained the entire time about supervision and management—now he wanted to see if he could do it better. When he went after an acting captain position (his department didn't have lieutenants), management debated long and hard about promoting him. He had been so critical of his supervisors that they were baffled about why he wanted to become part of a group he had openly ridiculed and despised. His chief's interview was grueling. The chief put it on the line. He would be watching Rob closely to see if he would be a leader, a problem solver, or a troublemaker.

Rob knew that being promoted to captain was the most challenging move a fire fighter could make. His responsibility would increase greatly: He would be accountable for the safety and behavior of his company in the station house and on scene. He would be responsible for the equipment and the apparatus they drove. He would be the one to maintain standards, set the tone, enforce general orders, and implement management policies, some of which he didn't support. At a fire, he would be accountable for forecasting fire behavior and keeping track of his company. Even off duty he would be held to a higher standard and could incur legal liability if something went wrong.

It was indeed a bigger job than Rob anticipated, and he felt humbled by it. He started studying again because he had to set an example for his company. If he didn't know something, how could he expect others to know more? If he wasn't in good shape, how could he demand that his company work out? If he didn't follow the rules, how could he discipline anyone else for violating standards?

His studying went far beyond the technical. He started reading books on leadership and management. He was very self-conscious, careful about what he said and what jokes he told. Fire fighters started coming to him to settle their squabbles. There were days when he felt more like a babysitter than a captain. He had tons of paperwork and meetings to attend on his days off. Discipline took up a lot of his time. He was especially uncomfortable when he had to discipline people he'd known for years, folks he considered his friends. There were days when he couldn't believe that he'd traded the best job in the world for this. Men and women who had been his friends were happy for him, but he noticed they sometimes became quiet when he walked into a room. He felt they were watching their step when they were around him, which often made him feel sad and isolated.

While the young fire fighters presented a challenge—there were so few fires to fight that he feared the younger folks were weak in basic fire-fighting skills and had little concept of how dangerous the job could be—motivating the veterans, some of whom were burned out, was an even tougher job.

Some days he felt trapped between "incompetent dinosaurs and incompetent newbies." At other times he grimaced inwardly because he thought he sounded like his hard-driving father, liberal with criticism and stingy with praise. It was an unpleasant insight. He laughed at himself for thinking like a manager. He had to admit it: things looked a lot different from this angle.

Managers in fire departments face stress unlike anything they ever faced in a field emergency. In all but the smallest communities or at the most extraordinary events, managers, particularly chiefs, rarely fight fires or respond to rescues. Instead they fight unions, budgets, city councils, city managers, and public opinion. The buck stops with them. When something goes wrong, they are held accountable. Their responsibility is immense.

"Ready, fire, aim" may work on the fireground, but not in organizational management. Once fire fighters move beyond the comfort and insularity of the firehouse, they are in uncharted territory. At this level, the tools they need are very different from the ones they are used to. The job has become less physical and more mental, less tactical and more organizational, less collegial and more political. Hardly anyone is prepared for this, neither fire fighter nor family.

When a chief's job opened up in a nearby community, Rob jumped for it. By now he had been a battalion commander for several years. He hadn't really liked the job. In some ways he had less power and influence over the troops than he did as a station captain. When the rank and file were angry at the chief, they were angry at him as well. After he enforced one unpopular management decision, several fire fighters stopped talking to him for a month. There was endless paperwork and numberless committee meetings, including mind-numbing sessions with the city council that lasted well into the night. With his workload and extra meetings he saw his wife and children less and less. He felt as if he had no where to go but up.

Two years after he became chief, there was an explosion in an industrial park in his jurisdiction. Toxic fumes filled the air and nearby residents had to be evacuated. There was major property damage at the site, but no injuries or loss of life. All the residents were permitted to return home within hours of the incident.

The search for villains began immediately and most of it landed on the fire department and public works. Rob stood in front of a series of town hall meetings, where he was the target of anger and insult. Everyday he and his department read in the newspapers about how they had failed the community. There was fighting among department heads, accusations were hurled from within and outside city hall.

Rob's wife was shocked and angry to read terrible things about her husband. More than anyone she knew how hard he worked and how much he cared. She tried to comfort him by telling him he had done the best he could under the circumstances, but he was not easily consoled. He felt he had let the community down and exposed his fire fighters and his fellow department heads to criticism from the public and the city council. It was agonizing to see himself and his colleagues pilloried in the press and to know that the source of some of the negative publicity came from disgruntled fire fighters in his department. It was the most difficult period in Rob's career as chief. The only thing worse was when he had to tell the family of a fallen fire fighter that their husband and father had died of a heart attack in the line of duty.

THE SEVENTH RUNG:
SELF-PRESERVATION ON THE ROAD TO RETIREMENT

Remember Chad, the 60-year-old fire fighter I mentioned at the beginning of this chapter? I ran into him on the street not long ago and we stopped to talk. He told me he was still having fun, although he was feeling burned out by dead bodies and auto wrecks. Mostly he felt physically compromised, especially when he compared himself to the younger fire fighters who were brimming with enthusiasm and energy. His back hurt and his knees ached. An old shoulder injury flared up every now and then. Senior citizens in nursing homes didn't look as old to him as they used to. He still worked out and was in better shape than others his age, but he wasn't bouncing back as rapidly after strenuous calls or sleepless nights.

No one ever said anything to him, but he sensed that the younger members of the crew were trying to do the heavy lifting and give him a break. He didn't want to be a burden, but more than that he didn't want to jeopardize himself or anyone else by being slow to respond. Whenever he could he shared his knowledge and years of experience with the new folks, and he made a point of mentoring one young fire fighter from every recruit class. These were very gratifying experiences.

But the fire service had changed. As much as Chad loved the young guys, he had less and less in common with them. They had a different mindset and he thought they lacked the dedication, persistence, and patience fire fighters his age once had. Young people didn't seem to appreciate their good fortune. As far as he was concerned, most of these kids with no college were lucky not to be picking lettuce or working as roofers. Still, they expected things to be handed to them, like promotions and special assignments.

Looking into the future Chad had two concerns. On the one hand, he couldn't imagine not being part of the fire service. He was apprehensive about losing so much comradeship and fraternity. He wasn't worried about having too little to do; he still had his side business and he looked after his grandkids. But he was worried about spending too much time with his wife, who had already warned him she wouldn't tolerate him laying on the couch watching daytime soaps or doing crossword puzzles, especially while she was still working.

Chad is a realist. "I don't kid myself," he said. "Once I leave, nobody's gonna remember me." He'd gotten some good advice from other retirees who told him, "If you come back to visit, don't stay more than five minutes. You won't know anybody and they won't know you."

"I don't want to be like Roger," he said, referring to another fire fighter who had retired two years earlier, "and sit in a lawn chair in front of my local firehouse drinking cocktails at noon."

Chad wanted what we all want: to retire while he still had the stamina to take trips abroad and to play with his grandchildren. He seemed more worried about this than he let on. There is a persistent firehouse myth that fire fighters don't live long after they retire. In fact, the opposite might be true: some actuarial studies show that fire fighters and police officers may actually live longer than other employees covered by their same retirement systems.

Chad never smoked, he watched his weight, and he always wore his SCBA gear when fighting fires. Still he was concerned. A friend of his caught a minor fire late in his career, inhaled some unknown toxin, developed lung problems, and died soon after retiring. With the finish line in sight, Chad didn't want to get hurt. Physical health was not his only consideration. He worried about carrying a "duffel bag of bad memories" with him into retirement. We all have slide carousels that revolve inside our heads. Chad had accumulated a lot of gory slides along with the good ones. He didn't want to add any more.

About 10 years ago Chad moved to a slower house that took fewer calls. Later, when an opening came up in the fire prevention bureau, he took it. It meant working a 40-hour week, but it got him off the line for a few years. Chad and his wife are good examples of how families can think ahead and mutually plan their way to an active retirement. Most couples won't arrive in the same place at the same time, or even have the same needs in terms of how to spend their time. Retirement is a big change and a big opportunity. Give yourselves ample time to anticipate and prepare for the practical and psychological consequences.

Tips for Career Management

- Plan ahead. Families who do fare better.
- Don't make any large purchases while in the academy and on probation. That only increases your stress.
- Determine early on what success and gratification mean to you and your mate. How do money, prestige, status, time together, and so on affect your definition of success?
- Establish mutual goals early in life that don't rely on promotion or overtime pay. Write up a family plan with realistic, achievable, and manageable goals for five-year increments from now through retirement. Begin investigating the realities of your financial situation and projecting your future economic needs against your future income. Discuss your mutual expectations.
- Save money from Year 1. Avoid living beyond your means or confusing material accumulation with genuine satisfaction. Create a back-up plan in case of injury.
- Don't put all your eggs in the fire service basket. Develop hobbies, interests, and friendships outside of work. They will help when the going gets rough or when you retire.
- Fire fighters: Consider earning a college degree; it is "insurance" in case you are injured on the job and it gives you more options when you retire. Many departments pay for it and there is usually time between alarms to study.
- Fire fighters: Choose your department carefully. Consider things like pace, commute time, affordable housing, opportunities beyond promotion, how employees are treated by management, and how the department is regarded in the community. Don't just apply because your uncle works there and the pay is good. Choosing a department is a long-term commitment with long-term outcomes. Spend some time hanging out. Talk with your family because they will share the consequences of your choices.
- Resist peer pressure when it runs against your standards. Houses and shifts have their own personalities and cultures. Find one that supports your best interests.
- Aim to live and retire in optimal health. Plan how you will grow old on the job. Pace yourself and stay fit. Identify those

(continued from previous page)

professional opportunities and career paths that will accommodate and challenge you as you age physically and mentally. Waiting until the last minute doesn't work.

- Consider consulting your Employee Assistance Program (EAP), chaplain, or peer support service to discuss any bad images or memories you have retained. Try to leave them behind before you retire.

CHAPTER 5

Emergency Medical Services
False Alarms and Frequent Fliers

> ... 80–90% of what we do in EMS is render compassionate
> care and resolve nonemergent conditions for our patients. The
> number of patients we bring back from the dead in a given
> year can be counted on our fingers and toes. But the
> number of times we give dextrose, bandage the forehead
> of a urine-soaked alcoholic fall victim or immobilize an
> elderly patient's fractured hip is almost uncountable.
> —A.J. HEIGHTMAN, Editor,
> *Journal of Emergency Medical Services*

I am visiting a firehouse located in the busy downtown area of a
large city in the Northeast. The department is staffed with 450
fire fighters. They run 12,000–14,000 fire calls per year and
39,000 medical calls—a pretty typical ratio. Today's my day to
ride with the medics. It's late morning and already hot as blazes.

I'll be riding with Rex, a veteran fire fighter/paramedic with
21 years' experience, and a rookie named Newman. (It is only
later in the day that I realize that "Newman" is slang for "rookie"
and all the Newmans I meet that day aren't related.) Rex used to
be an electrical contractor. He keeps his license up to date and
takes an occasional job when it suits him. He likes being busy and
working a "fast house." Good thing, because we're going to go all
day without a stop, which is typical for this part of town. We are
on "the wrong side of the tracks": government-subsidized hous-

ing projects, strip malls, light industry, and urban blight. My guess is that the fire fighters and fire fighter/paramedics who work here don't live anywhere close.

I've chosen to spend an entire day on the medic van because it's the best way I know to learn about what people really do in their work as opposed to what they might say they do. It's hard for families to get accurate information about what it's like to be a paramedic. For one thing, many paramedics don't like to talk about their work; some of it is too tragic to share with family, some of it too routinized to be interesting, and some of it too difficult to revisit. Frequently, they just want to think about something else for a while.

This doesn't satisfy a concerned family or help them understand why their fire fighter/paramedic seems moody or tired. It would be great if every family could ride along for a shift or two. But since this isn't practical, I decided to keep a log of this day's events and share it with my readers. Bearing in mind that the types of calls and the call volume vary from department to department, my objective was to capture the general pace, tempo, and "feel" of EMS work so that families can get a picture of what fire fighter/paramedics deal with on an "ordinary" day and why they may or may not need to talk about work when they get home.

- **11:30 A.M.:** A man has had a seizure and is lying unconscious on the sidewalk. In his pocket is a wad of money and a psychiatrist's business card, but no other identification.

We load him in the back of the medic van which is an old relic, creaky and hot. The medics are worried that the patient is going to "blow" (have a major seizure). They have to work fast without any information about his medical condition or what diseases he may carry. They're guessing drug overdose, so they give him a shot of Narcan, a narcotic antagonist that must be administered slowly or the patient will wake up in a highly combative state. Our guy doesn't react.

Rex turns off the air conditioner so the crew can hear better. They are monitoring the patient's heart rate, lungs, and blood pressure. They can't get his airway open, so they insert a breathing tube down his throat and then run a line of saline solution into his veins—all of this while we are bumping along the city streets. I'm the only one with her seat belt fastened.

Rex is still worried that the patient is going to have a seizure. Just in case, they turn him on his side so that if he does he won't inhale his own vomit. We pull into the hospital and Rex and Newman make a seamless transition into the emergency room (ER). Soon 11 people are working on the patient. Newman is crammed in a corner holding the IV bag while the hospital sets up it's own irrigation systems. The patient is catheterized through his penis. He vomits.

Someone takes the patient's temperature, which registers 108.5 degrees. This man is baking from the inside out and by all rights should be dead. By now the ER staff is fully in charge and the patient is hooked up to a ventilator. His prognosis is not good.

The pace changes abruptly as we move from the choreo-graphed chaos of the emergency room to a tiny report-writing room that has two computers, two chairs, a vending machine, and a table with a residue of sticky soda. Rex writes what will be the first of many reports detailing patient information, insurance cov-erage, time spent, miles driven, medicines and medical supplies fully and partially used. While Rex writes his report his radio crackles continuously with calls and the large double doors to the ER bang open repeatedly as other rescue squads wheel in the city's unfortunate and often most difficult patients.

Newman looks to be in his twenties. He's single and having a good time. He loves the money, the schedule, and all the time off. When I ask what stresses him about his work he has a ready list: "b.s." calls from people who don't take care of themselves and should; cops who dump "psycho" cases on paramedics because they're too "lazy" to handle the calls themselves; insufficient time to "nap, eat, or read" between calls; and meaningless chores as-signed by his captain and designed only, in Newman's estimation, to impress the chief. His responses seem typical of the Generation X'ers about whom veteran fire fighters complain.

• **1:00 P.M.:** As soon as the reports are complete, we are dis-patched to the home of a woman who is having trouble breathing. She lives in a tiny house in a run-down neighborhood. She is seated in the main room with four other women and three small children sprawled in front of the TV. One of the women lights a cigarette, seemingly oblivious to the effect the smoke may have on the patient who is struggling to catch her breath.

Rex gives the patient a pill. There is an brief angry exchange between her and another woman who is slow to get up and get her a glass of water. There are other outbursts as the women slap and yell at the children, who yell back.

Rex tries to persuade the patient to go to the hospital and teases her gently, saying she knows she'll wind up there later tonight. He doesn't mention that she will probably wake one of the paramedics to take her. He is easygoing and kind. He finally gets her to smile, but he can't get her to leave the house.

- **1:45 P.M.:** As we leave this patient we are dispatched to the home of a sick child. We can't find the address the dispatcher has given us. Each intersection is a challenge: drivers are seemingly struck dumb by the lights and sirens, or else they ignore them totally. We finally find the house, far from where we were originally sent. Rex and Newman are not happy with the dispatcher.

The patient is a feverish seven-year-old boy. He has recently been treated for a stomach infection and his symptoms suggest that the infection has returned. The child's mother is calm and prepared, having organized all her son's insurance forms and identification cards in a large purse—it appears there have been many such emergencies in her child's life. We load the boy and his mom into the ambulance and drive, without lights or sirens, to the local pediatric ER. Clearly the little boy is ill, but his condition is not urgent.

When I ask Rex why Mom called an ambulance, he tells me that some people don't know if they need to go to a hospital and call the paramedics to help them decide. Sometimes they erroneously believe they'll be seen sooner and taken more seriously if they arrive in the medic van. Rex says this without judgment.

- **4:00 P.M.:** We've been on the go since 11:30 and haven't had lunch. We're rummaging through the refrigerator at the station when another call comes in: an asthmatic is in distress. We slap some tuna salad on bread and run, sandwich in hand, to the rig. The patient is a man in his early twenties. He and his roommate are both massively overweight. Standing side by side they fill all the available space in their tiny living room. Both are dressed in hip-hop style: they are wearing baggy black clothes and have bandanas tied over their long, braided, shoulder-length hair.

Our patient, though he looks tough to me, is truly scared and making no effort to hide it. He tells Rex he feels like he's drowning. We take off in a hurry and Rex starts an IV—again, not an easy task in a moving vehicle. He says it took him four years to get the hang of it. One bad bump and the consequences for Rex or the patient could be dire. In a poor neighborhood like this, the rate of HIV and hepatitis is high. Many of Rex's coworkers have tested positive for hepatitis and tuberculosis (TB). He says it "comes with the territory."

Our patient had run out of medication and money at the same time. He has no medical insurance, no car, and he lives in housing that may well exacerbate his condition. We roll in, Code 3 (with lights and siren) toward the hospital. Along with thousands of other EMS units across the country, we are stopping up holes in a health care system that has failed the poor. It is a wonder that Rex and all the other paramedics aren't overwhelmed by the hopelessness of it all.

Everyday in the United States three people under 25 will die from AIDS, six children will commit suicide, 13 will be victims of homicide, and 8,500 will be reported as abused or neglected. Four hundred and thirty-four babies will be born to mothers who have had no prenatal care, nearly 2,000 will have no health insurance, and 2,500 will be born into poverty. Obesity, which is associated with serious health problems, has risen to epidemic proportions in the United States. This is a big hole to fill.

• 6:45 P.M.: We have just returned from patiently reassuring the mother of a newborn that her baby has indigestion, not some serious illness. Dinner is being served—pork chops, salad, corn, mashed potatoes, home-baked biscuits, and cool ice tea—all of which we leave behind when we are again summoned at 7:00 P.M. Newman slides down the pole, I run down the stairs, and Rex disappears without a word. His EMS tour is over and he gets to spend his remaining 12 hours working as a fire fighter. This department rotates their medics so they can get some rest.

Brad is driving. There's been a multiple car accident on the freeway with two victims. The accident victims are not badly hurt, but they are both in jeopardy due to their ages and chronic medical conditions. Between the two of them they suffer from coronary heart disease, diabetes, multiple sclerosis, obesity, and cancer. A second van arrives and gingerly removes one of the injured and takes him away. We transport the other, who is tethered to a backboard with his neck stabilized, deposit him at the nearest hospital, and head for home.

• 8:00 P.M.: As we drive into the apparatus bay we are dispatched again. There's no time to get out of the rig—we simply roll in one door and out the other. We have a hit-and-run accident. The injured driver is still in the driver's seat, crying. Brad tries to get her out of the car, but she weighs nearly 500 pounds. and can't be moved until additional help arrives.

Once on board the ambulance she asks Newman for some pain pills. She is crying miserably and complaining of pain in her back. He politely refuses, saying she needs to wait until a doctor can examine her. She is quiet for the rest of the trip. At the hospital Brad and Newman seem certain that her pain is bogus and she is naively hoping to get an insurance settlement.

• 9:30 P.M.: We have been back in the house for 20 minutes when the "brass (alarm bell) hits." A man with a gun is running around an apartment complex and we are asked to stand by in case there are shooting victims. By the time we arrive, the gunman has fled, but there are a dozen or so residents gathered in a parking lot screaming and yelling at two police officers, who appear very irritated with everyone. Two women have been hit in the face by the gunman, someone everyone knows, but neither has sustained any serious injuries. The hysteria seems to build with time, each woman reinforcing the other. We leave the cops to settle things down.

• 10:45 P.M.: It's been about an hour, the longest break of the day, when we are deployed to a local hotel to respond to a medical emergency involving a fire captain who appears to be having a heart attack. The mood is intense from the moment the call comes in: no joking, no sarcasm, no small talk. Everyone is focused on getting there as fast as possible.

Compared to the call we just made, this scene is eerily quiet. Everyone is moving quickly and soundlessly around the room, rendering some kind of medical assistance. They are plainly scared. This is one of their own, so no one wants to make a mistake. The gurney arrives and true to emergency responder culture— helpers are supposed to give help but not need it themselves—the stricken captain protests that he can walk to the ambulance unassisted. Clearly, he can't. He is very sick and will spend days in the cardiac care unit and then months at home recovering.

ALL GRIT, NO GLORY

Fires are fought in the open in front of people who have for eons been fascinated with fire and those who fight it. But the business of EMS is usually conducted behind closed doors. And when it is not, it evokes more anxiety than applause from a public that is both repelled and fascinated by the possibility that one day it could be them, or a loved one, lying on the sidewalk, covered by a plastic tarp.

In a profession that regards physical risk as a badge of courage, there are no badges for performing cardiopulmonary resuscitation (CPR) on a baby who has stopped breathing in his crib, or for telling the horrified parents that their child is truly dead and cannot be revived. There's little recognition for comforting the down-and-out, the lonely, the frightened, the aged, the homeless, and the addicted. There are no badges for treating people, regardless of their social status or stigma, with respect and dignity.

It is not that EMS is entirely without physical risk; fatigue, ergonomic injuries, and ambulance transport are major hazards. And EMS can be quite stressful emotionally and psychologically, something fire fighter/paramedics and their families need to anticipate and plan for.

Many fire fighter/paramedics complain that, compared to fire fighters, their jobs are more exhausting and less satisfying. They say they have less time to recuperate between calls, and they cite the strain of feeling responsible for the lives of the seriously ill and injured on a daily basis. On the other hand, they get paid more, have more education—sometimes subsidized by their departments—a more varied career path, and more opportunities to be of service to the community and make a difference in people's lives. Whether the added stress is offset by these factors is an ongoing debate. However you stand on the issue, the provision of medical care is part of the modern fire service and touches every fire fighter one way or another.

HOW EMS BECAME PART OF THE FIRE SERVICE

Medical response has been an occasional part of the U.S. fire service since after World War II when it became evident that Army medics, who were not physicians, were saving lives under the worst of conditions. Around 1969, the TV series *Emergency* raised the profile of fire fighter/paramedics and popularized the idea that fire departments could deliver quality medical care in record time. Until then, most fire fighters were only certified to administer advanced first aid.

The need has been phenomenal. Medical calls now account for 60–80% of all fire department calls for service. In 2002, for example, public fire departments in the United States responded to 12,903,000 medical aid calls, but only to 1,687,500 fire calls. While we do not know in hard numbers how many fire fighters run medical calls, we do know that the majority of large and small departments in the United States offer some level of EMS and most, but not all states, require fire fighters to be certified as emergency medical technicians (EMTs).

One consequence of expanding services from fire suppression to medical response has been that the public contact that fire fighter/paramedics have is more intimate and more emotional, placing them at greater risk for secondary traumatic stress or vicarious traumatization. *Secondary traumatic stress* refers to the emotional reactions experienced by people who have witnessed a scene of exceptional mental or physical stress, usually involving death or grave injury. It is amplified by feelings of failure, helplessness, fear, horror, or identification with the victim. For example, many fire fighter/paramedics who respond to a baby who has

81

stopped breathing have tiny children of their own. The parents' agony and helplessness thus hit close to home.

Exceptionally disturbing incidents have a way of stacking up, filling the spaces on the slide carousel in our heads. For a more complete discussion about the range of trauma, how it affects fire fighters, fire fighter/paramedics, and their families, and what to do about it, see Chapters 10 and 11. The material in this section is limited to describing some specific stressors associated with EMS.

Merger Madness

Before he became a fire fighter, Kenny was a paramedic working for a private ambulance company. When his company merged with the local fire department, he had to crosstrain as a fire fighter at the same time the fire fighters were being certified as EMTs or paramedics (see below for an explanation of how they differ). No one was happy. The fire fighters complained that they had signed on to fight fire and wanted nothing to do with medical calls, and the paramedics complained that they didn't want to be fire fighters and had never intended to be. Kenny was personally terrified of fire and it took a lot out of him to get through the fire academy.

When the merger first occurred there was a lot of distrust. Each group was convinced that the other would never be competent in their new roles. Most of the resentment has died down in Kenny's department, as it has elsewhere, although Kenny occasionally hears fire fighters criticize the paramedics for their firefighting skills and vice versa. What gets his goat is when fire fighter/paramedics are called "prima donnas" and told not to complain about how much their medical run volume exceeds the fire suppression runs because they get extra pay.

Historically, the deepest resentments stemmed from the suspicion that these mergers were forced on fire departments by outsiders whose primary goal was saving money, not community safety. This is likely an oversimplification of a very complex balancing act between fiscal reality and community need. There are benefits from incorporating emergency medical care into the fire service, not the least of which is that in most cities citizens can expect faster, more efficient, and more economical responses to medical emergencies from their fire departments than they can from private ambulance companies. Furthermore, the fire fighter/paramedic crews who show up are stable entities who have trained and worked together as a team and are accountable to a clearly defined command structure.

TRAINING AND CERTIFICATION

Fire fighters provide emergency medical care at two different levels of responsibility. EMTs provide basic life support (BLS), meaning that they can conduct an initial assessment of a victim's airway, breathing, and circulatory systems; administer basic first aid, CPR, defibrillation, and oxygen therapy; control bleeding; provide basic medical aid for illnesses, poisonings, injuries, and childbirth; and transport patients to the hospital.

Regulations vary from place to place, which is a source of continuous bureaucratic stress for the EMS service. California, for example, has 58 counties, each with a separate agency regulating EMS operations. Fifty-eight separate regulatory bodies makes for conflict, confusion, and a lot of red tape that other professionals, such as teachers and psychologists, don't face because they are regulated by a single statewide agency. So while there is a lot of variation, generally speaking, EMTs need approximately 160 hours (about six months) of on-the-job training and must pass both a written exam and a skills test. They are required to recertify every two years, which means they take additional skills and knowledge tests and complete a specified number of hours of continuing education.

Advanced life support (ALS) is provided by fire fighter/ paramedics who perform all of the basic services plus do advanced airway management such as intubation (forcing a breathing tube down the patient's throat), do advanced cardiac monitoring, run IV bags, and administer drug therapy. In addition, they're responsible for the safety of their crew and any bystanders. They need the skills and knowledge to make fast medical assessments, set priorities, make decisions, complete documentation, act as the patient's advocate, and help the crew restock the van and return to service quickly. Paramedics have EMT certification plus two years and nearly 2,000 hours of classroom training, hospital observation, and supervised field experience. They are required to recertify every two years, pass a skills test, and complete 60-plus hours of continuing education. Studying for these tests—whether you're a paramedic or an EMT—is stressful and takes time away from the family.

ALS ambulances are rolling emergency rooms and pharmacies. They carry a "ton" of supplies, all of which must be precisely stowed so they can be quickly found and then later accounted for. Failure to be able to do so can result in liability and possible administrative or criminal penalties. Here's just a partial list of the supplies for which paramedics are responsible: cardiac monitors, defibrillators, airway kits for conscious and unconscious victims, laryngoscopes and tubes in adult and pediatric sizes, forceps to remove obstructions in adult and pediatric sizes, CO_2 detectors, suction catheters, hand-held nebulizers for asthmatics, and pulse oximeters. They also carry rubber gloves, IV bags with two kinds of needles, Neo-Synephrine, xylocaine, epinephrine, lidocaine, dextrose, adenose, glucagon, Narcan, morphine, dopamine, atropine, sodium bicarbonate, bretylium, Lasix, Benadryl, Valium, and nitroglycerin. Taking care of all this stuff and all these people can spill over to the home in different ways.

STRESS

It is the call volume that gets to people. In some departments, you can sit around for months waiting for a good fire, but in many places medical emergencies are everyday occurrences and paramedics rarely get to sleep through the night. Incidents involving kids are the worst. Next hardest are the abuse cases, be they children or old people. It's hard for those who have dedicated their lives to helping others to see how much harm people can intentionally inflict on innocent victims and each other. So much of the wrenching despair that paramedics see is preventable, which makes it all the more difficult to accept.

Rex, the paramedic I rode with, complained that his former wife hadn't appreciated the chaos and the pace of his work and never gave him time to unwind. She would greet him at the door with demands, wanting him to take her places or talk about her day. She was a schoolteacher, and from her perspective Rex had a "cushy" job. I only heard his side of the story, of course, but I could see firsthand that his job is anything but cushy. When I asked him why she knew so little about the day-to-day reality of his job, he admitted that he didn't talk much about what he did and he never invited her to visit the station or go on a ride with him.

This is a problem for almost all emergency workers and their families. So much of what they see is too awful to talk about. How does a fire fighter tell her family about the teenager who hung himself from a rafter in the basement? And should she? Do they need to know? Sometimes it's easier to joke around with fellow paramedics—in the privacy of the ambulance or the station—about whether the hanging was a "Q," with tongue hanging out at an angle, or an "A," with tongue hanging straight down.

I have no idea if Rex made a unilateral decision that his wife needed to be shielded from the grim realities of his work, or if he was trying to avoid talking about it because he didn't want to revisit work in his head. It's a mistake to assume that families can't or won't understand, or to make a unilateral decision that they should be protected from knowing what happens at work. Families may not want or need to hear all the gory details, but they do want to be included in their loved one's circle of confidantes, and to be trusted enough to be part of their life away from home. Rex's wife may not have been at the scene, but she could understand universal human emotions like grief, frustration, and helplessness. And she could probably read Rex's nonverbal behavior and know when he had a bad day.

EMS workers have a tendency to manage their feelings, not just with humor, but by emphasizing the medical or clinical aspects of a call over the emotional ones. Like humor, this works some of the time for some of the people. There was an awful accident up in the hills. Two young men, ushers at a wedding, were speeding along a narrow country road in a convertible sports car, still dressed in their tuxedos, chugging on bottles of wedding champagne. The driver miscalculated a turn and drove off the road. Both young men were killed instantly. The driver's chest was crushed and his passenger was gruesomely impaled on a tree branch that went right through his head.

For days, Polaroid photos of the impaled victim circulated throughout the fire station and were posted on bulletin boards. There was a lot of joking and clinical discussion about entry and exit wounds. This kind of behavior is often hard for non-emergency responders and families to understand. It seems cruel and insensitive. But it is a common way for fire fighter/paramedics to handle horrific events by depersonalizing the victim and pushing away the certain knowledge that one minute you can be on top of the world and one millisecond later you are dead.

High-Stakes Habits

Terry has been a fire fighter/paramedic for years and he drives his wife, Jill, nuts trying to keep everything as shipshape at home as he keeps it at work. This is an impossible goal because they have three small children who leave their toys around, like most kids do.

Terry's need for orderliness creates a lot of discord. Jill knows his job is stressful, but she doesn't know how many dreadful calls he has gone on involving children because he doesn't tell her. Instead he comes home and yells when he finds toys on the steps or cabinet doors slightly ajar. His obsessive concern with order gives him some momentary relief from the tension he brings home from work, but it is a temporary fix at best. He knows he can't keep his kids safe by lining up all the Tupperware by size. Worse still, he is starting to alienate his children and turn his home, which should be a sanctuary from work, into a place of friction.

Sonny, on the other hand, is a slob and he makes no bones about it. He is tired of keeping things clean and perfectly organized at work. When he's home, he drops everything where it falls and leaves it for his wife to pick up. When she does, he complains she's "too tidy." This is a family joke. Because Sonny isn't edgy or critical, their different standards of neatness are rarely more than a minor irritation between them.

The Golden Hour

The clock starts ticking at the time of injury or illness. After what is called the "golden hour," most patients' chances of survival go downhill rapidly. So the pressure is on as soon as a call comes in:

pressure to get to the scene, to stabilize the patient, and to leave as quickly as possible. Frequently, there's only time enough to "load and go," giving whatever treatment you can in the ambulance as you're barreling toward the hospital.

Occasionally, there's not even a "golden minute" and emergency responders have to help resuscitate the victim on the spot, get him breathing or get his heart going. This can be rough on fire fighters, especially those who don't do it very often.

Taking Things Personally

Dick is a volunteer fire fighter. Like many volunteers, he lives in a rural area with few medical services. The nearest hospital emergency room is 20 minutes away by helicopter. The call came in during dinner: an 82-year-old man named Howard had collapsed, probably from a heart attack. His wife told the dispatcher she didn't know how long her husband had been lying on the floor of their bedroom.

Dick jumped up from the table and ran to his car. He was relieved that he didn't know Howard or his wife. As a volunteer fire fighter/EMT in a small town, he knew a lot of his patients personally. When he arrived, Howard wasn't breathing. Dick and Ben, another volunteer, began CPR, trying to keep Howard alive until the fire engine from the neighboring county arrived with a defibrillator. It was the only choice they had, but it wasn't an easy one. CPR broke every brittle rib in Howard's chest and he died anyway. Dick felt horrible and vowed he would never again perform CPR on such an old person.

"Routine" calls such as CPR can leave a persistent, psychological aftermath. Howard's death stuck with Dick and he worried that he would be unable to stop staff from performing CPR on his frail, elderly mother when she was hospitalized years later with a terminal illness.

Winning or Losing

Winning or losing is often how fire fighters and paramedics look at their work. Keeping score can be discouraging because there are relatively few dramatic "saves" in EMS, especially in "sudden death" or immediate threat-to-life situations when the "golden hour" shrinks to just four golden minutes. After four minutes the survival rate drops to 20%; after eight minutes most immediate threats to life are fatal and the survival rate drops to 1%.

Harvey told me he was a religious man and that he ultimately put life and death "in the Lord's hands." He believes his role as a paramedic is not to play God, but to act as a medium between God and the patient. His mindset keeps things in perspective and cuts down on ruthless second guessing and self-blame. The idea that a fire fighter/paramedic should be able to save everyone is a terrible burden, because many times, as Dick has found out, you can do your best and the patient dies anyway.

The more paramedics believe they have control over the outcome of a call, the more psychological stress they may experience, especially if the outcome is negative. The reasoning is flawed, but compelling: if I have control over what happens and my patient dies, I must have done something wrong. Conversely, a paramedic who thinks he or she has little influence over a patient's medical condition might feel discouraged from the outset and give up sooner. Often there is no black and white, only shades of gray, leaving plenty of room for painful second guessing.

Jack and Sandy, both fire fighter/paramedics, almost came to blows over coding (declaring dead) the victim of a hit-and-run. The victim was a young woman on her way to work. Her head had been crushed and there was visible brain matter. Jack said she was dead. Sandy wouldn't accept this verdict. The patient had a very weak pulse. For Sandy, that was enough to keep trying everything at his disposal. Jack declared that the victim's pulse was a biological sputter that meant nothing. Sandy screamed that he didn't get into this business to pronounce people dead, that was the coroner's job and he was going to keep at it until the coroner told him to stop. He was ultimately overruled and he ruminated about it for months. He thought seriously about quitting the program and getting back on the engine.

Intimate Strangers

Imagine what Dick felt while performing CPR on Howard. He heard Howard's ribs cracking, felt with his own hands how thin and frail he was, heard his wife crying in the background, saw every bristle on his face, inhaled the scents of coffee and old clothes, and saw pictures of his children and grandchildren on the night stand next to his bed. This is intimacy. While such experiences do not always have long-term negative consequences, they do, as they did for Dick, have "velcro" and can stick around in the mind, for better or for worse.

Most fire fighter/paramedics have an album of such events in their heads. They can bring each scene to life with a moment's notice. Certainly not all the scenes are bad; some may be downright funny and some truly rewarding. My point is that EMS brings fire fighters into frequent intimate contact with the public under conditions of significant stress, when they are physiologically in high drive, geared up to absorb and catalogue sensory experiences. Too many significant experiences with too little time to recover can, without intervention, lead to *burnout*: a state of apathy in which fire fighter/paramedics protect themselves against stress by adopting an uncaring attitude.

On the other hand, intimacy with strangers can lead to lifelong bonding. The massacre at Columbine High School is a good example of what often happens when fire fighters and victims have prolonged contact under highly stressful circumstances. It was a horrific scene: gunshots and explosions could be heard everywhere. It was impossible to distinguish police gunfire from the shooters' gunfire and no one knew where the shooters were. When it was over, 15 were dead and 24 were injured. Afterward, fire fighters turned toward, not away from, the victims. They sold T-shirts, pins, and posters, donating the proceeds to a fund for healing. One collected flowers from the memorial and made potpourri bundles to pass out to graduating seniors. Almost all the fire fighter/paramedics kept in touch with their young patients. They had become, as one paramedic described it, "lifelong friends."

Burnout

Fire fighter/paramedics have a tendency to let their dedication get in the way of their own well-being. That's what happened to Charles. He loved helping people and believed he did a good job, but he was constantly angry and upset with his new fire chief because he felt the new chief didn't value or support the EMS function as much as the previous chief had. Charles had disagreement after disagreement with the chief over equipment and protocols. He believed the public was being misled about EMS availability and response time. His frustration built to such a point that he had a meltdown on the job and demanded that he be returned to fire suppression even though he knew that his department required that paramedics give six months' notice before transferring. His request was denied, which led to months of painful wrangling and grievances.

Charles was a single man with no one at home to give him some feedback on his state of mind. Had he talked about his problems to someone else, he might have accepted the fact that he would never agree with the new chief and his policies and that it was futile to try. He might also have acknowledged that he had had years of being a successful paramedic, but that everything comes to an end and it's best to leave on a high note when you can.

One of the best approaches to burnout is variety. Of course, in small departments, there may not be other job opportunities. Finding new interests, outlets, or activities outside of the job helps. So does counseling (see Chapter 14) and stress management (see Resources).

Frequent Fliers

Some of the most irritating calls in EMS are the "frequent fliers," people who repeatedly abuse the system in pursuit of their own agendas. They don't care if they wake paramedics out of a sound sleep, and they don't care about tying up a paramedic crew that might be needed elsewhere for a real emergency. Some of these calls can be funny, but over time they can also contribute to burnout and bitterness.

I am bunking in a firehouse on a freezing cold evening. We've been out on three calls and only got to sleep at 3:30 A.M. At 6:00 A.M. the lights and the alarm go off again and we are dispatched to a single-vehicle collision. As we pull up to the vehicle, which is parked on the shoulder of a two-lane highway, I hear Herman, the paramedic say, "Oh, dear mother of God!" I expect to see bodies sticking through the windshield. Instead, there are two women sitting quietly in their car. One has a tiny cut on her ankle, origin unknown. The other has no injuries but wants to tell us what happened in excruciating detail while we are standing on the road in the snow and the sleet. Their car has a miniscule dent on the rear quarter panel, where they hit a fence.

This is the second time this evening that Herman has responded to a call from these two women, although they never acknowledge this. They called 911 earlier because one woman's boyfriend was refusing to take his medication and they wanted the paramedics to insist he do so. Herman treats these patients respectfully, masking his irritation and contempt. As soon as a highway patrol officer arrives we leave. "Idiots," Herman snarls to himself, "retards."

We are asleep barely one hour when the alarm and lights are activated again. There is an unconscious female at a local hotel. "What a hummer," Herman says. It turns out that an employee fell asleep on the job and feigned unconsciousness to avoid being disciplined. But Herman and the EMT know what to do: they expose the "lazy faker" by applying pressure to the bed of her fingernail and giving her a serious pinch on the muscles at the back of her neck. This is standard protocol for determining unconsciousness, but I can tell they enjoyed this payback for waking them out of a sound sleep for nothing.

The next call simply produces groans. It's Dirk, a local drunk who regularly calls 911. What he really wants is a ride to the liquor store, which is closer to the Veterans' hospital than it is to his house. He has no qualms about faking a seizure or a fall in order to get a lift. When he calls, the paramedics have to respond, and so will the emergency room staff.

Responsibility

Terry, a very young fire fighter/EMT wants his family to understand how close he feels to other fire fighters, how much he loves his work, how hard he works, and how stressful the work is, particularly because it's unpredictable and he never knows what will happen next.

No sooner has he said this, than the bells go off. An elderly woman is having some kind of attack, but is apparently able to breathe. It is raining outside and we drive, with flashing lights and siren on, into an unfamiliar housing development. Our flashing lights bounce off the hood of the "squad," making it hard to see the house numbers in the rain. We make one or two wrong turns. Terry, who is driving, is getting increasingly tense as valuable minutes of the golden hour tick by. Mack, the paramedic, is trying to help, but he's having a hard time reading the map in a moving vehicle. Fortunately the callers are watching for us, blinking their house lights off and on.

We run into the house. There are six people in the living room. The elderly woman is sitting in a leather recliner. She appears dazed, her skin is yellow and dry. Her pulse registers at 35, 40 beats below normal. Terry runs for the gurney, and comes back dripping wet from the rain, apologizing for tracking water on the rug.

The elderly woman refuses to go to the hospital. She has stomach cancer, breast cancer, and last week she had an angioplasty, a procedure that opens blocked blood vessels to the heart. As she talks, color returns to her face and she appears weak, but increasingly alert. She explains to Mack that she had simply forgotten to take her blood pressure medications on time and her blood pressure dropped precipitously. This happens regularly. Usually she can wait it out watching TV. But tonight she and her husband had dinner guests and she was busy cooking.

Mack checks her pressure again. Now it is better. Even so, he insists on taking the patient to the hospital for a more thorough examination. The patient still refuses. Mack calls the hospital and consults with the doctor on duty, who agrees that the best course of action is to transport the patient to the ER. The patient is not impressed with the doctor's advice and signs a form refusing medical treatment.

Mack and Terry are clearly upset. Mack is certain the patient will get worse. Back at the firehouse he continues to fret. He feels responsible and worries that he should have been more insistent. In the win/lose world of emergency response, Mack feels as though he has lost. He doesn't have the luxury of seeing things from the patient's point of view. But when he considers the woman's age and multiple illnesses, he speculates that it may be preferable to die among friends than to die among strangers in a hospital, hooked up to machines and tubes. Reframing things from this angle seems to make him feel better.

Mack's concern is a good example of how fire fighter/EMTs and fire fighter/paramedics shoulder a steady stream of responsibility. They must do their work quickly and compassionately, under the worst of circumstances. Their patients are not always cooperative, grateful, honest, or clean. They make important decisions with minimal information, little time, and often not enough sleep. Everything they do or fail to do has consequences.

Tips for Dealing with EMS Stress

- Coping with stress requires many tools: exercise, hobbies, pleasant escapes, lighthearted distractions, long-range goals, a variety of interests and friends, comforting rituals, and philosophical or spiritual beliefs. As a couple, balance work with play. Take family trips, sign up for a cooking class, or buy a board game you can play together.
- Fire fighters: keep your spouses informed about your work lives, but only share as much information as she or he can tolerate. (You'll only know this by talking about the limits of her or his tolerance.) If you've had a bad shift and a sleepless night, say so.
- Social support from family *and* coworkers is absolutely essential in managing secondary traumatic stress. One study of 1,750 fire fighters and fire fighter/paramedics concluded that the more satisfied fire fighter/paramedics were with the social support they received at home and at work, the less they were bothered by recent critical incidents, sleep disturbance, and feelings of vulnerability. Approximately 80% of this survey sample were married, and on the whole reported high levels of satisfaction with support received at home.
- If you get queasy hearing about blood and gore, tell your spouse that details aren't important to you. They can, and maybe should, review the details with their coworkers. What

(cont.)

(*continued from previous page*)

you really want to ask is: "How are you feeling?", "What do you need now?", and "How can I help?"

- If your mate doesn't like to talk when he or she is stressed, find out what else you can do. Support comes in two categories: emotional and practical. Both are important and both make a difference. Find out if your fire fighter would like a back rub, time alone, a good meal, a funny video, and so on. Maybe you could pinch-hit by helping with the children's homework, driving your in-laws to the doctor, or paying the bills.
- Give your fire fighter a chance to shift gears and decompress after work. Try not to greet him or her with problems. Schedule a mutually good time to talk. Write it on the family calendar. Most emergency responders find it easier to keep scheduled dates than to make spontaneous plans.
- Get the facts: find out how much good sleep your loved one had the night before. Remember, it's hard to sleep deeply when anticipating that you might be awakened any moment, even if the alarm never goes off. Some psychologists think that there is considerably more stress when the annual EMS call volume falls below 200 or exceeds 600.
- If the department allows it, go on a ride-along/sleep-along. Just dropping by the firehouse at dinner time may not give you an accurate picture of the pace of the work.
- Be aware that not all stress results from line-of-duty incidents. In fact, most stress is organizational (see Chapter 6). On any given day your EMT/paramedic fire fighter can be mired in paperwork; overwhelmed with regulations; caught in a turf fight between local, state, and county EMS authorities; be the object of a bogus complaint by a patient who is trying to get out of paying the ambulance bill; or be frustrated by trying to keep up with changing requirements for recertification.

Organizational Stress

Fractures in the Fire Service

The fire service: 100 years of tradition,
unimpeded by progress. . . .
—ANONYMOUS

In order to understand what makes fire fighters tick, you have to know as much about the organizations in which they work as you do about the work they do. Families have a vested interest in this subject. Studies have shown that spouses can be vicariously affected by organizational stress and office politics as well as be resentful of the degree to which both intrude into family life. It's hard for families to get an objective or neutral view of organizational life, especially if the sole source of information is their fire fighter.

Howard told me he used to come home and complain to his family about how bad things were at work: administrators were egotistical and unfair, bad people got promoted while good people were disciplined, and so on. At first it felt good to blow off steam, but eventually it backfired. His wife and family developed such a negative attitude toward his department that he wound up having to defend himself and his department—which wasn't really as bad as he made it out to be. It's human nature to complain—public safety responders who are trained to look for what's wrong or might go wrong are especially vulnerable to this trait—but it gave Howard's family a distorted view of a job he really loved. Howard's advice to families? Take what you hear with a grain of salt.

Organizational stress affects everyone with a job. It's not unique to the fire service, although some characteristics of the service—the paramilitary structure or the living arrangements, for example—can make it worse or better. A professor of mine used to say, "There are no good organizations," and many days I'm inclined to agree with him. We rarely train people to anticipate or manage organizational stress, even though it's part of their day-to-day life. What helps to minimize organizational stress are realistic expectations; a skeptical, but not cynical, outlook; and the ability to stand back and take the long view of things.

When people talk about what creates stress for fire fighters they tend to think first about line-of-duty incidents like fires and rescues. But they would be wrong. Bureaucracies create stress and fire fighters work in highly structured bureaucracies. Bureaucratic or organizational stress routinely exceeds line-of-duty stress in studies of fire fighters and fire fighter/paramedics. In one study of nearly 2,000 fire fighters and fire fighter/paramedics, conflicts between labor and management were more robustly and consistently correlated with job dissatisfaction and poor work morale than were critical incidents. Only sleep disturbance had a higher correlation.

Over the years researchers from many countries have identified several sources of organizational stress, some of which affect career fire fighters more than volunteer fire fighters, and some of which affect both equally.

- Poor leadership, management, and supervision
- Conflicts between superiors and subordinates
- Inadequate training
- Promotions, limited career ladders, and seniority
- Poor policies and procedures
- Inadequate resources and equipment
- Personality conflicts with crew members/shift-mates
- Budget cuts and threatened reductions in force
- Politics

- Labor/management conflicts
- Race- and gender-based harassment and reverse discrimination

Let's take a look at how many of these organizational stressors play out.

POOR LEADERSHIP, MANAGEMENT, AND SUPERVISION

One of the biggest problems in the fire service is the lack of professionally trained managers and supervisors. It simply doesn't work to promote fire fighters on the basis of their technical skills or seniority and expect them to be as good at managing people as they are at managing events. Yet this is how leaders are often chosen. Studies show that the overall correlation between experience and leadership performance in the fire service is near zero. Retired assistant chief Dr. Carl Holmes describes the seniority system as "the most professional method on earth to measure how long people have worked for you. Otherwise, it isn't worth s——t!"

The further up the ladder you climb, the more you need to know how to lead others and solve complex problems. This is especially true for the company officer, who has the most contact with line staff. Unfortunately, people who are skilled working under pressure where decisions are made quickly in the worst of circumstances do not automatically possess the skills needed to manage people when the pressure is off. Seventy to eighty percent of fire fighters' service time is spent in nonemergency tasks—most career fire fighters spend an average of 22 hours anticipating alarms and only two hours responding to them.

Untrained leaders rarely have the opportunity to get the training they need, so they do the best they can with what they have. But sometimes their best isn't good enough. For example, untrained supervisors may not know the difference between being *authoritarian* (bossy and intimidating) and being *authoritative* (knowledgeable and leaderly). Or they may be too timid, failing to confront bad behavior because they don't want to risk alienating anyone. This can get more complicated if they are represented by the same union as the rank and file, or if they can't depend on their human resource departments to back them up when disciplining an insubordinate employee.

A colleague of mine was standing in front of a fire station talking to the fire chief when a fire fighter walked past. "Good morning, Al," the chief said, "how are you doing?" "None of your f——ing business," Al replied and walked on. "Poor Al," the chief confided, "he's upset with me because he didn't get the promotion he wanted. He'll get over it." And that was it. No discipline, no counseling, no consequences except those that spilled over to the fire fighters who overheard this exchange. The message they got was that it's okay to be disrespectful to the chief because you'll get away with it. And if you can be disrespectful to the chief, what's to stop you from being disrespectful to other superior staff, to each other, or to the public?

LABOR UNIONS: CAN'T LIVE WITH 'EM, CAN'T LIVE WITHOUT 'EM

Union activity is part of most fire fighters' lives. Volunteer fire fighters are represented by the National Volunteer Fire Council (NVFC) and paid fire fighters are represented by the International Association of Fire Fighters (IAFF), although one-third of the IAFF membership comes from volunteer departments. The IAFF is one of the 50 most powerful political action groups in the United States. It is not unusual for them to raise millions of dollars to support political candidates of their choice. They are highly organized and proactively seek to expand their influence by training members to seek political office.

Depending on who you talk to and where they work, the union is a blessing, a burden, or both. A lot depends on the local leadership. Union officials are proud of fighting for the health and safety of fire fighters. And they are determined to continue the fight, to keep on funding programs and initiating legal challenges against those who put money first and fire fighter safety second.

I'm talking to Ray, a gray and grizzled guy just months short of retirement. He is the informal historian for his department. "In the old days," Ray tells me, "before the union arrived, working in this place was like living in a totalitarian country. It was a dictatorship. The old chief ran everything military-style. He had absolute power; we didn't even know we had rights. He would make us wash his wife's car as well as his own. We were constantly rolling and restocking hose, washing the rigs, and polishing brass. Didn't make any difference if we only moved the trucks five feet, we had to wash the wheels and the floor or we got disciplined. There was a lot of politics and favoritism. If the chief liked you or you were a relative, you got promoted. Once when I threatened to quit and go to another department, the chief refused to give me a reference and said he was going to accuse me of stealing. He was so mad he threw a paperweight at me. It was oppressive. He put on a good face to the city council, so nobody believed us when we complained. Then the union came in and put a stop to it."

No question about it, unions stop a lot of egregious behavior and fight fiercely to protect the line fire fighter. But sometimes the union leadership is out of touch with its members. A fiscal crisis hit one moderate-sized city and looked like it might negatively affect public safety funding. The rank and file in the fire department felt unfairly vilified by the media and abandoned by their management, who seemed not to be fighting hard enough against cuts in the fire department's budget. Worst of all, they felt hoodwinked by a small but vocal group of union leaders who decided on their own to send inflammatory letters to the citizens and to threaten withdrawing their support from city council members they had previously endorsed. These were unwise moves. The community was furious, the council was up in arms, and the rank and file felt their union leadership had unilaterally made things worse for everyone.

It's true that unions take pride in enforcing collective bargaining rules that ensure that fire fighters are properly paid and fairly treated by their departments. Creating and retaining jobs for fire fighters is a high priority. In fact, conflicts over reductions in force have been known to galvanize fire fighters into action, some of which is endorsed by the union and some of which is done vigilante-style, anonymously and in the dark. Once antagonized, normally harmonious fire fighters can be spurred to take a range of aggressive steps to get what they want: political protest, strikes, community organizing, letter-writing campaigns, smear campaigns, poor-faith contract negotiations, extortion, theft, and even arson.

Union critics accuse both the locals and the national union of being short-sighted and self-serving by placing membership needs before the community it pretends to support and by overstating danger and safety issues for the sole purpose of retaining jobs. They say the membership is "held together by unhappiness" and officials are elected on the strength of their ability to "object to everyone and everything." Still, one might wonder how much worse things would be if the union wasn't around?

Sometimes the issues are incredibly complex. Francis had been appointed as the academy training coordinator. His predecessor had left the academy in shambles: understaffed, over budget, and out of compliance with various guidelines. Francis turned the situation around, but in the process created a lot of enemies, including the city manager, who removed Francis from the job, accusing him of misappropriation of funds, dereliction of duty, and fraudulent use of overtime.

The next six years were a nightmare for Francis. He was found innocent of the criminal charges but guilty of administrative wrongdoing, for which he was suspended for two months without pay. He filed a lawsuit against the city and after months of legal wrangling won his case. (He only wished the media had paid as much attention to his exoneration as they had to his indictment.) The cost for his victories? Fifty thousand dollars in union funds and $60,000 in personal savings.

Francis's elation was short-lived because his department refused to reinstate him at the academy and he was forced to take a position in the prevention bureau. When he again turned to his local for help, it balked. The union president was worried that supporting Francis might anger the powers that be, especially the city manager, and jeopardize upcoming union negotiations. As a loyal union member Francis understood that his union couldn't sacrifice the well-being of the whole for the interests of one person. Still, he wondered if the union president had another agenda. So many fire fighters held Francis in high esteem for fighting back and winning his case that Francis was now publicly considering running for union president in the next election.

VOLUNTEERS VERSUS CAREERISTS

> ... not a Fire happens in this Town, but soon after ... the
> Place is crowded by active Men of different Ages,
> Professions and Titles; who, as of one Mind and Rank,
> apply themselves with all Vigilance and Resolution,
> according to their Abilities, to the hard Work of conquering
> the increasing Fire. ... They do it not for Sake of Reward
> of Money or Fame: There is no Provision of either made
> for them. ... Ye Men of Courage, Industry, and Goodness,
> continue thus in well doing; ... it will be thought by every
> good Man who sees your Performances; here are brave
> Men, Men of Spirit and Humanity, good Citizens, or
> Neighbors, capable and worthy of civil Society, and the
> Enjoyment of a happy Government.
> —BENJAMIN FRANKLIN, founder of the
> first volunteer fire-fighting brigade, 1773

Two hundred and thirty years after Benjamin Franklin wrote his famous essay "Brave Men at Fires" we still depend upon a volunteer force of nearly 800,000 men and women to rescue us, give us emergency medical care, and put out our fires. Volunteers comprise 73% of the U.S. fire service. The majority of fire departments are fully volunteer. They protect approximately 23% of the population of the United States, principally those living in communities of fewer than 10,000. In 2002, 67 volunteer fire fighters died in the line of duty. Volunteer fire fighting, rescue, and EMS entails risk in the way few other volunteer opportunities do.

As volunteerism decreases, the trend is toward creating combination departments where volunteer and paid fire fighters work side by side. The transition from an all-volunteer or all-career department to a combination department, or the consolidation of several separate volunteer or career departments, is part of the modernization of the fire service. And like other modernization in the fire service, it can mean trouble. Retired chief, author, and fire service historian Ronny J. Coleman writes that all fire departments will experience conflict as they move from an all-volunteer staff to incorporating paid personnel. In some instances the transition has been handled professionally, but in other cases it's been a "dogfight."

There are many reasons for the conflict. Volunteer fire fighters have great personal investments in their departments. It's a time-consuming service; many volunteers regularly contribute 20–25 hours a week for years on end. In addition to emergency responses, they spend time training, fundraising, attending meetings, taking care of equipment, and handling administrative details.

Volunteers have deep ties to their communities and are threatened by the prospect of losing their autonomy as nonprofit organizations and coming under the control of a governmental bureaucracy, even when they stand to gain from subsidized training and funding for better equipment. Fire chiefs in particular are apprehensive and taxed by the complications raised by consolidation, not the least of which is working with formal collective bargaining procedures that come with career fire fighters who are members of the IAFF.

I often joke that perception, not possession, is nine-tenths of the law. When departments combine there is a lot of mutual eyeballing. Career and volunteer fire fighters tend to have generally positive attitudes about themselves and negative attitudes about the other. Each group thinks the other is getting a better deal for less effort. Volunteers may assume the paid fire fighters are in it solely for the money, job security, and devotion to their second jobs. Paid fire fighters may believe that volunteers are insufficiently trained, less competent, and reluctant to take orders from careerists—meaning they may not integrate easily into the nationally standardized fireground command structure. They worry about volunteers being less physically fit and are concerned about being given reliable backup. With little social interaction between the two groups, these speculations are rarely tested. This is especially true when careerists and volunteers are trained separately and held to different performance standards.

As far as Shelley, a fire fighter/paramedic, is concerned, volunteers in her department are only in it for the fun and they just get in the way. She has a list of complaints: Volunteers don't clean up after themselves. They expect the paid folks to do the grunt work while they parade around in their turnout gear driving fancy apparatus with the sirens blaring. They don't keep current with training, they are too excitable, and they make poor decisions in a crisis. She thinks a paid person should be in charge of all emergency incidents, even when the volunteer is equally capable or holds a higher rank. Fortunately, from her point of view, she's able to avoid most of the volunteers because she works days and they work nights and weekends.

The Two-Hatter Controversy

The IAFF has an official policy that prohibits union members from volunteering in jurisdictions where there are paid fire fighters represented by the union. This has come to be known as the "Two-Hatter Controversy," which in some parts of the country is a very contentious issue.

Career fire fighters want to volunteer for many reasons. For Andy, returning to volunteer in the small rural community where he had learned the ropes was enlightened self-interest. It gave him a chance to socialize with his friends and neighbors and it was an opportunity to "catch" more fires and sharpen his skills on his days off. He was therefore shocked when he received a letter from the president of his local declaring that he was in violation of the IAFF constitution and by-laws. His affiliation with a "rival organization" was considered "misconduct" and he was given 60 days to "disaffiliate" himself from his volunteer fire department or turn in his union membership card.

Andy didn't want to quit the union, lose his union benefits, and alienate his fellow union members. On the other hand, he had deep ties to his volunteer department and he didn't want to leave it short-handed. He wondered why it was anyone's business what he did in his spare time.

He listened to the arguments on both sides. Andy knew that his union was working diligently to protect the community as well as his health, safety, benefits, and wages. He felt badly being told that what he thought was a good deed was "negatively impacting the growth and prosperity" of his fellow fire fighters, something he would never do. He was confused. The only time he heard of volunteers replacing paid fire fighters involved some career fire fighters who worked 8:00–5:00 shifts and then volunteered in their same departments in the evening. Andy could understand why the union objected to that.

Andy decided to talk to Doug, one of the veteran fire fighters in his career department. He knew Doug had recently quit his long-time volunteer position. Doug told him he thought the issues went way beyond job security. He believed that his community had grown large enough to merit round-the-clock paid services. He felt certain that his neighbors overestimated how quickly volunteers could respond to an emergency and underestimated how many fire fighters were needed to effectively and safely handle a crisis. He also worried that he was jeopardizing his own safety showing up at a fire with only one or two other available volunteers. His family was concerned because they knew that career fire fighters who are hurt or die in the line of duty while volunteering will not get the same benefits, pensions, or worker's compensation settlements to which they're entitled on their paid jobs.

Andy thought this all over. It was true that volunteering exposed fire fighters to injuries. On the other hand, nearly half his department moonlighted in nonunion construction or automotive repair, jobs that entailed physically dangerous work and hazardous materials. One of his coworkers had fallen off a roof he was fixing and was on disability for six months with a badly broken leg. Another one broke his hip training for a triathlon.

Andy was sympathetic to the concerns of his volunteer department. Everyone there was afraid that if the IAFF bylaws were enforced they would lose so many volunteers that his small community would be in danger and might be forced to hire paid fire fighters it could ill afford. The community had other pressing needs to consider when doling out limited funds. His chief was irate. Wasn't Andy being a good citizen by answering President Bush's call for Americans to volunteer in their communities after the tragedies of September 11th? As I write this, Andy is leaning toward regretfully resigning his volunteer fire fighter position and finding another way he can make a contribution to his community.

IN-HOUSE CONFLICTS: WHO MOVED THE TOASTER?

Marriage and family life are a challenge. It's amazing that two or more human beings with different backgrounds, values, biological and sexual requirements, communication styles, sleeping patterns, and eating habits can form a working partnership that meets everyone's needs most of the time. And I'm talking about intentional families, people who choose to live under the same roof.

Think of how much more difficult it can be when the family you live with is unintentional. Fire fighters live in work families that are artifacts of assignment, seniority, and luck. The ordinary strains and irritations of living together are magnified by working in tight-knit crews under less-than-optimal conditions. The intense degree to which fire fighters depend on each other in the field heightens the significance of even trivial interpersonal disagreements—disagreements that often can't be worked out informally because most fire departments are structured in a rigid, paramilitary fashion.

How you get along with the people you live with for part of the week can make or break your career, especially when you're stuck on a small crew and can't get out. When you're happy with your crew mates the days fly by, when you're not happy it can feel like being in prison.

Conflicts can arise between fire fighters of the same rank. Frank and Murray worked EMS together. They were dispatched to a restaurant where a patron complained of a racing heart. After Frank and Murray made their preliminary assessment, the patient said he felt better and wanted to drive himself home. Frank agreed, but Murray wanted to take him to the hospital. Frank and the patient outvoted Murray. That was the end of the call, except that Murray couldn't stop thinking about it. He felt that he was right and that Frank was lazy and taking chances.

Murray didn't much like Frank anyway because he was the kind of guy who never cleaned up after himself in the kitchen. Murray stewed about the incident all the rest of the shift and finally confided his frustration to another medic named Jake, who also had issues with Frank. Jake told someone else on another shift and that person told the EMS coordinator. Frank had a lot of friends on the other shift, and before Murray knew what was happening there was a "cold war" between the shifts. The situation grew progressively worse; Murray and Jake were Caucasian and Frank and his friends were Latinos. Frank described the experience as a "runaway train." It didn't take long before the disagreement over one clinical procedure was rumored to be a racially motivated attempt to get Frank in trouble.

The next few months were very uncomfortable. Frank took every chance to lash out at Murray who was by now sorry he ever said anything to Jake. Murray's wife listened patiently and tried to help. But after several months she grew tired of listening to Murray go round and round about this. She felt she had reached the limits of her ability to help and suggested that Murray consult with the department psychologist. It was a good idea. The psychologist coached Murray about ways to approach Frank and gave him some ideas about how to settle their conflicts. Murray waited until the passage of time seemed to have softened the tension a little bit and then he told Frank he wanted to talk in the hopes that they could air their disagreements and put things behind them. Frank agreed. As angry as he was, he too was tired of the friction. Talking helped. Though neither will become the other's best friend, Frank is convinced that Murray's intentions were not racially motivated and Murray has learned that he could and should speak directly to Frank when there is a problem.

Tips for Dealing with Organizational Stress

- Organizational stress is part of the territory, but don't let it occupy all your conversations. Try to find some balance and perspective. Don't get swept up in the anger or the fear.
- Organizational issues are intense and draining. Family members may need someone who is not involved to support them while they are supporting their fire fighter.
- Organizational stress provokes strong emotions. Don't be a target for frustration. If your fire fighter is displacing frustration or anger at the organization onto you or your family, steer him or her back to the real problem. If he or she can't use you as a sounding board, a compassionate confidant, or a fellow problem solver, it is time to end the discussion.
- My colleague Dr. Alexis Artwohl thinks that 60–70% of all employee stress is caused by poor supervisors. If fire fighters don't accept this inevitability they can feel betrayed and

---

(continued from previous page)

abused, and may choose inappropriate means to deal with the situation. Don't personalize things. Everyone gets a poor supervisor or even a poor crew from time to time. Better to take the long view and wait it out until you can make a change.

- Fire fighters: pick your battles carefully. In a conflict between an individual and an organization, the individual is usually at a disadvantage, even with union support. Save your energy and anger for the "big ones," if and when they occur.
- Know your legal rights and ask for help when you need it, but understand that legal victories are costly and sometimes hollow.
- Never let anyone put you up to a fight that isn't your own or that you don't believe in.
- Know your representation. When you have a problem, find representatives who do not have an ax to grind, a personal agenda to forward, or an ego to feed. Seek out people who will firmly represent your interests while remaining open to mediation or negotiated settlements.
- Learn and practice good interpersonal skills. You'll need them as much with coworkers as community members. Too many conflicts escalate only because the people involved didn't know how to express themselves well, control their emotions, or apologize.

CHAPTER 7

Diversity

... the world has changed ... this is not a
dirt trail anymore. It's a six-lane highway.
—ROBERT DEMMONS,
retired San Francisco fire chief

I'm at a large conference featuring, among other topics, workshops on leadership skills for a diverse fire service. The day is over
and I've been invited to join several fire fighters for a cocktail in
the bar. I'm the only female present. Everyone is gracious and hospitable, including a young battalion chief who is sitting next to
me. He's the only manager at the table. The group is talking about
diversity and sharing stories of how they recruit and retain female
fire fighters. The battalion chief describes himself as a progressive
role model for caring and courtesy. He tells the group that his department is very professional and that he personally will not stand
for any disrespect, especially in the presence of women: a modest
goal since his department is all white and 99% male.

By the second round of drinks, the conversation has moved to
a discussion of food, weight, and body shape. It hasn't been sexual, but it is getting close. At this point the battalion chief tells a
story about a beautiful woman he dated a few years ago. He describes her as having huge breasts and then gestures with his
hands to demonstrate just how large her breasts were. When the
relationship broke up his battallion chief—whom he depicts as a
caring guy with a great sense of humor—came by the firehouse
and presented him with a consolation gift that he describes—

108

using his hands again—as an anatomically correct doll. By this time everyone is laughing but me.

I'm not laughing because I'm upset and irritated. I'm a guest at this conference; I don't want to insult my newfound companions, nor do I want to embarrass the battalion chief in front of the group. On the other hand, I'm wondering what happened to all that talk about respect? Could he be so eager to be liked that he would jettison all his principles to be one of the guys? Is he a hypocrite? Am I being set up or am I being super-sensitive?

My discomfort will be familiar to anyone who has ever been a member of a statistical minority. It's isolating. When you are one among many nothing is what it seems, every comment has a double meaning, and every interaction feels like a test whether it is or it isn't. It makes no difference *why* you are a numerical minority—race, age, religion, body size, politics, gender, or social status—you feel different, and people treat you differently. Being one among many adds significant strain to the already challenging job of fire fighting.

I tell the battalion chief that in California his former chief would be in a heap of trouble for giving him a present like that. He is astonished and irritated. "Are you kidding?," he asks, "Do you mean that he could get into trouble for trying to cheer me up?" It is obvious that he is unclear on the concept. I then ask if he hasn't discussed hostile work environments and sexual harassment at this conference. "No," he barks and withdraws into moody silence. A moment later he abruptly gets up from the table and leaves the room without a word. Ten minutes later, he still hasn't returned.

The fire fighters at the table seem embarrassed. One of them jokes that the battalion chief probably spends most of his conference time playing tennis instead of going to workshops. Another comments that he can dish it out but can't take it. Somebody else calls him a hypocrite. Two people ask me if I am going to write about this incident in my book. When I ask, "Do you think I should?", they answer "Yes" in unison.

It's a paradox. The fire service has an honorable history of risking lives to help those who cannot help themselves regardless of race or gender. At the same time it has a long, shameful tradition of exclusivity. The good news is that in the past three or four decades minority males have made significant inroads into the profession. The bad news is that females have barely made it past the front door. Gay men are still in hiding.

There are approximately 275,000 career fire fighters in the United States, of whom nearly 84% are Caucasian, 12% are African American, 4% are Hispanic, and less than 1% are Native American or Asian. Women make up only 3% (about 6,100 positions), and the majority of them are Caucasian. Another 40,000 women work in the volunteer, paid-on-call, part-time, and seasonal sectors. (Sexual integration is even less advanced in the United Kingdom, where only 0.5% of paid fire fighters and 1.5% of volunteers are female.) The first woman chief of a career department was promoted in 1993. Eleven years later there are just 15 female chiefs running career or combination departments and several dozen in the volunteer service. Compared to other protective services, the fire service is lagging behind. Women constitute nearly 12% of law enforcement and nearly 15% of active-duty military.

THE CHALLENGES OF CHANGE

Numbers aren't everything. Once inside, minority males and women face a range of challenges beyond those inherent in just doing their jobs—not the least of which is trying to fit in where they may not be welcome. Unfortunately, fitting in or meeting standards even when they are equally applied does not solve all the problems that arise from diversification. To quote the authors of *A Handbook on Women in the Fire Service*, all of them current or former fire fighters, "Altering the identity of people in a fundamentally unaltered workplace can leave the door open to friction, miscommunication and a host of inequities" (p. 4).

Social change, even progressive social change, creates pain for everyone. Majority groups suffer considerable distress when they feel they and their families are being damaged by social changes beyond their control or blamed for social inequities they did not create. Their distress is real too and deserves attention.

PROTECTING THE IMAGE

So what is at stake for the majority fire fighter? His reputation, his self-esteem, and the persistent myth that only white males can be competent fire fighters. Fire fighting has always been viewed as the essence of masculinity. It has been long thought that being a woman and being a fire fighter are incompatible. Throughout history portraits, photos, and posters of fire fighters at work portrayed women and children as helpless victims to be rescued. Rescues of men are almost completely absent in the visual representations of fire fighting. An 1884 edition of *Fireman* magazine reprinted an article from the *New York Times* about a group of British college women who were eager to form a fire brigade to protect their campus. The *New York Times* condemned the venture on the grounds of modesty: "That the fire girls should actually ascend the ladders in full gaze of the public . . . while the fierce light of fire plays about their ankles is . . . unthinkable" (quoted in Cooper, 1995).

Likewise, a series of satiric prints titled *The Darktown Fire Brigade* (1885), issued by the famous printmakers Currier and Ives, portrayed black fire fighters as incompetent, disorganized, and "ape-like," according to art historian Robyn Cooper. The series was a mocking parallel to a realistically drawn series titled *The Life of a Fireman* that portrayed hardworking regimented teams of slim-hipped, broad-shouldered, white firemen and their incredible steam machines—machines universally referred to in the female gender. Was it only coincidence that Nathanial Currier was himself a volunteer fire fighter in New York City?

RACE AND GENDER

> . . . women will have a hard time becoming fire fighters to the extent that to be a fire fighter means to be a man. Men of color may find some aspects of fire fighter culture distasteful . . . but there is no inherent opposition between fire fighter identity and the identity of a man of color.
> —CAROL CHETKOVICH, *Real Heat*

Luis was hired after his community demanded that the fire department provide a bilingual speaker in every fire station. It was automatically assumed by the white fire fighters that he was an "affirmative action shoe-in" rather than a qualified fire fighter. Along with everything else he had to face as a rookie, he had to deal with white people's perceptions and their caustic comments. At one of his first stations a captain demanded to know how he got the job. This captain had an ax to grind because his two sons had been passed over for employment. "Well, sir," Luis replied, "I was picking crops in the field in Mexico when a recruiter stopped me and asked if I wanted to be a fire fighter. I said 'Sure,' and they hired me just like that. Any more questions?" Luis was fighting sarcasm with sarcasm. He would have much preferred to deal with his captain's concerns in a more direct and respectful manner, but his response stopped the stupid questions.

In most fire departments, paid or volunteer, the easiest person to be is a white guy. If a white guy makes a mistake, that's just him and most people tolerate it or cover his back. But if a minority male or any female makes a mistake, it is too often taken as confirmation that people of color or women can't do the work.

In studies of gender differences in fire fighter job stress, women reported significantly higher levels of coworker conflict and significantly higher concerns about making mistakes, having inadequate skills, being "perfect," and meeting standards. The researchers attributed the higher scores to two factors: women feel they are under scrutiny and that higher standards *are* being applied to their work. Women who are the first to be hired in their departments come under even greater pressure, knowing that if they're not successful, it will be harder for other women to be hired in the future.

Race also plays a part; while a majority of white women fire fighters surveyed by the Women in the Fire Service felt that they were treated differently and negatively because they were women, over 92% of the African American women felt this way! Gender is intertwined with race. Black women fire fighters can never separate the two or set either one aside. White women fire fighters rarely realize the privilege their race gives them, but it does count for something to have the potential to trade on racial and ethnic bonds with the majority.

All women are marginalized in similar ways in the fire service, but there are significant variations based on race. Take stereotyping, for example. Black women fire fighters are often stereotyped as loud, antagonistic, athletic, welfare recipients, and "beasts of burden" who can shoulder heavy loads and do more chores than others. While all fire service women have to prove themselves physically, white women are more often stereotyped as "fragile," and may struggle to counter that image by hiding their injuries and pushing beyond their limits. Sometimes they have to fight off subtle and blatant attempts to "protect" them from hard work. Black women rarely encounter such "chivalry," leading one researcher to conclude that "white women are challenged by underburdening, African American women by overburdening" (Yoder & Berendsen, 2001, p. 27).

Men of color often appreciate the plight of women fire fighters because they identify with their struggles to gain entry to the fire service. But they also frequently hold the same biases as majority males. In some instances they are relieved to no longer be the scrutinized statistical minority. They distance themselves from women's issues rather than risk being back in the line of fire.

Colleen, who is African American, was the first woman hired by her department, a distinction that resulted in more pain than honor. She was a single mother looking for a steady job with good benefits. It wasn't political for her and she wasn't trying to make a statement. Things were awful from day one. All the fire fighters resented her presence, but her primary tormentor was Ollie, the only other black fire fighter in her house.

Ollie was hostile, menacing, insulting, and totally uncooperative. Reasoning didn't help, being black together didn't help, appeals to his conscience didn't help. The more she tried, the worse it got. Colleen started to fear for her safety. Ollie had made it clear that she had better watch her back in a fire, because he wouldn't. She finally went to her lieutenant and told him about her concerns. Amazingly, he agreed with her and said, "Well, Colleen, I don't think he'll actually hurt you, but if you got in trouble I know he wouldn't help you." Even more amazing, he did nothing about it. He didn't transfer Colleen nor did he discipline Ollie.

Colleen's troubles with Ollie ultimately escalated into a

physical confrontation: he threatened to "kick her butt" and she grabbed an ax and swung at him until he backed off. It wasn't until the only black battalion chief in her department got wind of the situation that she was transferred to a different house, one where a supportive captain could be trusted to keep his eye on her.

Colleen's situation is not all that uncommon—and sadly things can get even worse. What happens when minority fire fighters, males and females, find swastikas and racial epithets painted on their lockers? When they are called names, jeopardized on the fireground, and shut out of training they need to do their jobs? Or when they are retaliated against for complaining?

What happens when women fire fighters are grabbed and fondled? When male fire fighters "accidentally" expose themselves in the bunk room? When they receive death threats on their answering machines or have their personal files stolen and released to the press? When they are subjected to watching pornographic videos in the firehouse, forced to listen to coworkers speculate about themselves or other women in base sexual terms, discover wet spots of semen in their bedrolls and peepholes in their dressing rooms? When they are forced to move refrigerators or heavy patients by themselves while other fire fighters stand around laughing. When they find human feces in their shower stalls and straight pins in their back pockets? When they are given the silent treatment or much much worse for speaking out about these offenses?

Actions like these go far beyond traditional firehouse pranks. Stopping them requires efforts far beyond individual responses. These are not rare occurrences: various studies indicate that between one-half and three-quarters of women surveyed in the career and volunteer services have experienced some of the offensive behaviors listed above.

SISTERS IN THE BROTHERHOOD

Fred Astaire was a great dancer, but Ginger Rogers danced backwards and in high heels.

—ANONYMOUS

It is hard for a woman to be acknowledged for her actions unless she makes a mistake. When a woman is hired or promoted, the usual gossip is that she got the job because of her gender, not because of her merit. Men need only be as good as each other. A woman fire fighter has to prove she is as good as any man and she has to do this at every rank. This has profound implications for her ability to perform her job safely.

Wendy is small by anyone's standards: five feet three inches tall and 115 pounds. Passing the physical agility test was very difficult for her, but she trained hard, carrying her 160-pound boyfriend up and down the stairs of their house. In the interview portion of the hiring process she was put on the spot and asked a question not posed to male applicants: "How would you feel about being the only female in this department?" She was prepared for this. "Ecstatic," she said. "I can't wait." Then she made a risky but plucky move and turned the tables on her interviewers. "How do you feel having me here? Are you going to change for me, because I won't change for you." She made this declaration without any real understanding of how much she was actually going to have to adapt.

Her first day at work was a media circus with all the attention on her. It was unwanted attention and she was fearful that the other new fire fighters, who were equally proud of themselves, would resent her and think she was conceited. She already knew she would have to prove herself to them all over again. She took a lot of ribbing and everyone called her "Ms. Movie Star," but by and large their teasing was good-humored. It helped that she was a tomboy as a child and grew up with a lot of males in her family.

A year and a half later she still doesn't know if her coworkers accept her. She finds them hard to read. She struggles with knowing when they are joking and when they are serious. And she thinks they find her equally hard to read: one minute she is a joke-telling prankster who can dish it out as well as take it, another minute she's crying about a dog that's been run over by a car. These subtle kinds of interactions create low-level strain and add another dimension to the self-consciousness most new fire fighters feel about their competency and their ability to fit in.

A firehouse is like a one-room cabin. People who may never before have associated with groups other than their own are now living together, spending 90% of their time in fire station activities. Men and women are sleeping in the same dorms and using the same bathrooms.

A variation of this holds true in the volunteer service, even though members come from the same community and tend to share the same ancestry. Volunteer firehouses often operate as the center of small-town or rural social life. When things don't work out for the newcomers, they can't easily transfer to another house or another department.

Janie couldn't get to first base with her fellow volunteers. They were disrespectful and laughed at her behind her back as she tried to learn how to be a fire fighter. One day she was out in the hot sun trying to start the chain saw, something she had never done before. Over and over again she pulled on the starter cord until her arm and her back ached and sweat and tears ran down her face. She wouldn't ask for help because she thought it would make her look even more helpless than she actually felt. No one offered to assist her or to show her what to do. Nobody cared that with a little help, some advice, and maybe some modifications in technique, Janie could become an asset instead of a joke. With volunteerism shrinking in the United States, volunteer fire departments should be thinking about how to get women to join rather than devising ways to keep them out or chase them away.

Few fire departments prepare their employees for dealing with diversity. A lot of training is simply superficial, a one-size-fits-all approach whose main purpose is to cover the department's legal obligations. Poorly designed training about diversity, sexual harassment, and discrimination only inflames the situation.

A common complaint about the presence of newcomers—females, in particular—is that they have eroded the closeness and playfulness male fire fighters enjoy and value. Jack, a white man with about seven years' experience, was very candid about his views. His department is one of the success stories, a place that actively and thoughtfully recruits and supports women and minorities. When his department first hired women Jack actually wondered if it was a stress test to see how much a person could take.

"The family feeling is gone," he said. "We have fewer things in common, fewer shared interests, and we don't hang out and help each other off duty as much as we used to. Before women got here we played around a lot more. But they made us stop tossing buckets of water on each other. I guess women found it too threatening and some guys were actually charged with assault."

Lawsuits

Lawsuits are a reality of modern society; they are painful for all involved, plaintiffs and defendants alike. Unfortunately, they sometimes represent the last and only way to bring about change in an intractable system. While it is difficult to find the exact numbers, the fire service has been inundated with lawsuits pertaining to race discrimination and gender bias in hiring and promotions, reverse discrimination, sexual harassment, hair-length policies, safety issues, and nepotism (issues of fairness arising from working with a relative or a spouse). Some of these issues are directly linked to changes in diversity. Hair policies have been based on the needs and styles of white men. Should women fire fighters be forced to cut their hair short? Is there a direct and provable connection to hair length and safety? Why would a department have rules against corn rows and braids before they hired any African Americans?

Some of these cases have or will wind up as consent decrees that may be in place for decades. *Consent decrees*—legally binding agreements supervised by court-appointed monitors—may get the ball rolling in terms of righting past inequities. On the other hand, they can cloud the issue. When women and ethnic minorities are hired under consent decrees, it is easy for majority fire fighters to question whether the new hires are truly qualified or whether they were hired under lowered standards devised to fill court-ordered mandates. The newcomers may also share these doubts, especially women who often internalize the belief that they cannot do the job as well as men.

THE BENEFITS OF INCLUSION

The benefits of inclusion extend beyond the right to fair and competitive access to meaningful work with status, security, and decent pay. Dr. Portia Rawles, a diversity consultant who was a fire fighter for 15 years, maintains that a diversified fire service will have greater creativity and a wider range of ideas and input. It will have improved problem solving resulting from a convergence of perspectives. There will be better service to all quarters of society and an appreciation for the commonalities of the human condition.

For example, women in the fire service may soften or counterbalance attitudes usually associated with male identity: rugged individualism, a stiff upper lip, extreme risk taking, and a go-it-alone, never-ask-for-help personality. All of these have been repeatedly implicated in substance abuse, posttraumatic stress disorder, emotional problems, deteriorating family relations, and a host of other cascading physical and psychological dysfunctions.

As 80% of all fire department calls are medical, women add to the range of comfort provided to female patients who may be embarrassed and uncomfortable being ill or naked in front of men. The same holds true for rape victims and victims of domestic abuse who might find the presence of females reassuring—as reassuring as a female fire fighter may find having a male coworker on scene when the abuser is still present.

The fact of the matter is that in work this hard, people need each other. In the video *Test of Courage: The Making of a Fire Fighter*, a Vietnamese-speaking fire fighter tells about being dispatched to a car fire. The driver and his passenger, both non-English-speaking Vietnamese, didn't want the fire department to put out the fire because they thought they had to pay for that service. The Vietnamese fire fighter was able to explain the problem to his crew and to reassure the victims that the fire suppression services were free. Who knows what kind of confusion and damage would have occurred if he hadn't been present—if his department didn't reflect its customer base?

Dennis, a paramedic, told me about going on a call to a Muslim family. When they were gathering information about the patient, one of his crew picked up a copy of the Koran to lean on while taking notes. The family was visibly disturbed. Dennis, recognizing the book and its sacred meaning, grabbed it and put it back. He apologized to the family and got the offending fire fighter out of the house before the situation escalated further. This incident occurred shortly after the events of 9/11 when fear and trepidation were sky-high in the Muslim American community.

ASSOCIATIONS AND ORGANIZATIONS

The attempt to achieve diversity in the fire service has generated a variety of associations and educational institutions devoted to the specific needs and interests of women and various minority groups. Sometimes these associations are seen as threats to the predominant labor organization and its locals. In fact, these specialized associations exist in part because some of those traditional locals have been slow to respond to the concerns of women and ethnic minorities.

Fire fighters' associations based on ethnicity and gender were first formed to deal with issues of fairness and equity on the job; they try to influence the fire service culture and correct historical inequities. But they also extend their reach well beyond these issues by going into their constituent communities as role models, seeking to inspire girls and children of color to imagine that they too can be fire fighters. These groups bring fire education into underserved areas, hold classes, and distribute fire safety literature in the language of the community they want to reach. And they exert political influence to provide quality emergency services where such services may not exist.

For example, a Native American is three times more likely to die in a fire than the average U.S. citizen. In many cases, tribal fire departments have been left out of their local emergency response systems. In response, tribal fire chiefs formed their own association to study the fire problems in Native American communities and work to improve existing fire protection, suppression, and life safety services. Some call this divisive, others call it leadership.

Luis, the Latino fire fighter I discussed earlier in this chapter, is a busy man. He juggles his loyalty and his time between the National Association of Hispanic Fire fighters, the Bomberos (a statewide organization), and the IAFF. When he first joined the department his local was controlled by a clique of "angry white men" who were fighting to retain control of the workforce. They seemed fearful that Hispanics and African American fire fighters were "taking over." Luis finds this laughable. He says that at the rate things are going, he'll be a great-grandfather before either men of color or women achieve any level of critical mass and influence within the fire service.

Luis had contemplated "defecting" from the IAFF but decided to stay because he believed the only way he could make change was to work within the system. But few people took him seriously or respected what he had to say. He got a jacket (reputation) for being vocal and active. Even his mother warned him that he was too "militant."

Luis lived with narrow-mindedness, arrogance, and inappropriate comments, but refused to be drawn into negative conversations, gossip, and name calling. When people insulted him or anyone else, he confronted them in private. He tried to stay focused on his own objectives. When he was shut out of training opportunities, as were many minorities at the time, he and others simply put together training of their own.

His persistence paid off and things are now very much better. The small clique that drove the union has retired or been silenced. His administration is supportive and "takes care of business" when it comes to issues affecting women and minorities.

Respect seems to be what it's all about. Luis doesn't need to be liked—he can separate who he is from the job he does. What he has fought for for himself and other minorities is equal access to fire service jobs, a chance to succeed, and respect as individuals, something many white men take for granted.

ADAPTING TO DIFFERENCES

When a woman shows that she is as tough and aggressive as a man, she may get a reputation for being castrating, pushy, or strident. She herself may feel less feminine as though she has to sacrifice who she really is to do the job she wants. She has to be masculine on the line but feminine in the firehouse, tough at work but nurturing at home. It seems to make little difference whether she is gay or straight.

Males and females are socialized differently and they come to any job with different strengths and weaknesses. When people are willing to help women succeed in the fire service these differences can be successfully accommodated without compromising accepted methods of safe fire fighting and rescue. After all, right-handed male fire fighters don't object to teaching left-handed male fire fighters how to tie knots differently. They don't reflexively complain that adapting procedures for the left-handers is "special treatment"—code words for lowering standards.

New techniques and technology designed to make the job easier and safer benefit everyone, not just women: lighter SCBA bottles, pullout steps or hydraulic racks, wheeled carts for moving heavy equipment, and pulleys for ladder halyards. One recently retired fire fighter told me that lighter equipment made his heavy work more manageable and actually extended his career.

Wendy and Pam set up a mentoring program for four recently hired women fire fighters. They themselves had had a hard time being the first women in their department and they wanted to make things easier for the newcomers. As they observed the rookies at work they noticed the women approached fires gingerly, carefully stepping over shrubs and flower beds. One of the first things Wendy and Pam did was give the women permission to step on the shrubs: this was not a time to appreciate or preserve the aesthetics of the fire scene, something women are socialized to do. None of the men needed to be told this.

Is it fair to judge how well women can do as fire fighters when they have to struggle just to get the equipment and protective gear that allows them to train and work safely and properly? Women are generally smaller than men; their hands are smaller and they have less upper-body strength. A 1995 survey of 500 female fire fighters found that only 39% had gear and uniforms that fit. And what they had they got only because they were willing to spend years fighting for it. How do you run in boots three sizes too large, breathe with SCBA masks that don't seal, see under a helmet that collides with your air tank, or use your hands in gloves that are too big?

FEMALE FIRE FIGHTERS AT HOME

Sometimes women fire fighters have even less support at home than they do on the job, even though home is where most of us get the comfort and reassurance we need. Connie is an Asian American fire fighter, the first in her traditional family and the first in her department. It's a joke that she's a "twofer" because when she was hired her department got to fill two minority slots: Asian and female.

Connie's husband, a business executive, was not at all enthusiastic about her job choice. It seemed like role reversal: Connie was doing dirty dangerous work and he was sitting behind a desk shuffling papers. Her father, especially, was dead set against her joining the fire service; from the moment she did, he began referring to her as his "son." Whenever she dropped by to visit he would ask her mother, "Is that my son at the door?" It was very hurtful, but Connie put up with it out of respect and the mistaken hope that her father would eventually stop. But one day she had had enough. When he asked once again "Is that my son?", she pulled off her T-shirt, stood in front of him in her brassiere, and yelled "I'm your daughter—your sons don't have breasts." It was a dramatic moment, but it ended his sarcasm. He never again referred to her as his son.

Many fire service women complain that the men they meet are intimidated by them. They're not secure enough to date women who are tougher, stronger, and do more important work than they do. They can't relate comfortably to women who are assertive and self-confident. It's not uncommon for male fighters' wives to be jealous of women fire fighters and anxious about sleeping arrangements in the firehouse. But it goes the other way too, many men are uncomfortable being with a woman who spends a lot of time on the job or as a volunteer surrounded by men or actually living with them. No wonder many women wind up dating or marrying other fire fighters (see Chapter 13).

Chrissy's parents and her boyfriend, Les, a carpenter, think she's going through a phase. She was caught in a backdraft and suffered steam burns on her arms. It was so hot part of her hood melted. She called Les and her parents from the hospital. Their responses were not comforting. Her mother asked if Chrissy was ready now to get a "real job." And Les said, "I hope you're done with this," implying that Chrissy couldn't handle the danger. What she was done with, she retorted, was him.

They didn't talk for several days and when they did Les admitted that he was truly frightened for Chrissy's safety. He also confessed for the first time that he took a lot of ribbing on his job and from his friends. Sometimes his buddies kidded him about

Chrissy being a guy in drag. Other times they teased him about her having a thing for guys with "long hoses." Chrissy was sympathetic and they talked about what he could do or say to blow them off, but she held firm. She wasn't going to quit her job because he couldn't stand up to his buddies.

Domestic Life

Despite gains made in equality between men and women—today's men are much more involved in family life than their fathers were—studies still find that women continue to spend significantly more time than men caring for their families and that they are more likely to adjust their work lives to their families' needs. In the fire service this can backfire because the prevalent point of view is that when a male fire fighter stays home with a sick child he is a hero, but when a woman fire fighter stays home it's because she can't get her life together.

Some people consider childcare to be the fire service's number-one challenge. Until it is resolved, the fire service cannot be truly hospitable to women and many men. Career fire fighters work in 24-hour shifts and their children need round-the-clock care. Volunteers and career fire fighters are both subject to emergency calls and callbacks. Fire fighter couples and single parents are especially affected. Thirty-two percent of all women fire fighters are married or involved with other fire fighters; 11% are or have been single parents.

Most families need two incomes just to keep up. Many of us live far away from our extended families and some of us are "sandwiched" between raising young children and caring for elderly parents.

Worrying about your children while working increases stress on parents of both sexes and diminishes their effectiveness. Increased stress is also the reason some women may leave jobs they have worked very hard to get. Lois was raising three kids by herself. She worked two nine-hour and two 15-hour shifts at a very busy firehouse. She had endured a contentious divorce. Her husband, a police officer, fought her for custody, claiming that working 24-hour shifts made her an unfit parent. He lost, but he left Lois in a tight spot. She didn't want to give up a good-paying job she loved. On the other hand, she knew that her ex had her under surveillance. Any slip in her childcare arrangements and he would take her back to court.

Dependable childcare was so hard to find that Lois ultimately hired some help and started her own 24-hour daycare at home so that she had a place to leave her kids. She feels guilty that her children had to do so much for themselves and grow up so fast, but she also thinks the challenges they faced as a family helped them to grow up as independent, confident, and trustworthy teens. She's proud of them and they are proud of her.

GAYS AND LESBIANS IN THE FIRE SERVICE

In 2002, President George W. Bush signed the Mychal Judge Act that expanded the categories of people who qualify as beneficiaries and are eligible to collect $250,000 in federal death benefits guaranteed to public safety officers killed in the line of duty. The expanded categories now include siblings and same-sex or opposite-sex domestic partners. Prior to this bill only parents, spouses, and children were eligible to collect. The bill is named after Father Mychal Judge, a New York City Fire Department chaplain who was killed during the September 11th terrorist attacks on the World Trade Center. It's been widely reported that Father Judge was gay.

It took an enormous tragedy to acknowledge the presence of homosexual fire fighters. Gay men, especially, threaten the status quo. Like women, gay men are stereotyped by some as lacking courage and loyalty. When they act bravely and competently they threaten the cherished notion that only "manly men" can be fire fighters. They also threaten the social order of the firehouse, which, as one gay fire fighter told me, is a "grab-ass" locker-room fest. For straight men, the presence of openly gay men sexualizes ordinary but intimate activities like sleeping and showering. This happens even when the gay guys are in committed relationships and wouldn't presume to make a move on a coworker, especially a heterosexual coworker.

The unknown consequences of being openly gay are powerful. Even fire fighters who lived through the horror of the collapse of the twin towers on September 11th were fearful of coming out in public. It's not an easy decision. Gays and lesbians don't choose their sexual orientation, they are likely born with it. But they can choose to be public or private about their orientation because it is not overtly obvious in the way race and gender are. This is a highly individual decision with immense consequences and legal overtones. No one can or should make that decision for another person.

Bryan had known all his life that he was gay. What he wanted was a "normal" life. He didn't want to hide who he was, nor did he want to fight discrimination on a daily basis. And he wanted a family. He joined the fire service at 23 and that pretty much clinched it; he loved his job and he knew for certain that he'd be miserable as an openly gay fire fighter. He had no role models, no companions, and no support for being different. He got married and had children. He loved being a father. It was only after he divorced and came out to his wife and his now-grown kids that he came out in public by appearing, in uniform, at a high-school career day for gay teens. It was an important event for Bryan, who felt strongly that gay youth need role models. A reporter spotted him and the next day Bryan was in the headlines.

When he returned to the firehouse where he'd worked for many years, he naively expected to be treated the same—after all, he was still the same person. His crew mates gave him the silent treatment; no one asked him about himself or even expressed an opinion. There were sniggers in the background and meaningful glances across the kitchen table. Six months later, Bryan transferred to another location. His former wife and his children were able to accept him as he was, his former shift-mates could not.

Lesbian fire fighters seem to be less threatening to the status quo. In the fire service, women are more frequently stigmatized for their gender than for their sexual orientation. Still, homophobia and sex discrimination are linked together. Women have lost jobs simply because someone thought a strong assertive woman must be a lesbian. Myrna is 35 and never married. She is a wildland fire fighter, and straight. But it's been hard finding a man who would put up with her being away for weeks at a time. She is strong and muscular with short hair and a boyish walk. Her sexuality is constantly in question and the subject of many coffee table conversations despite telling others that she isn't gay. She lives and works in a community that is very religious. Being labeled a lesbian is not idle name calling: it could cost her her part-time job coaching girl's soccer, jeopardize her personal safety, and embarrass her friends and family. Myrna worries about this a lot. For a long time it kept her from getting together with other women fire fighters or attending conferences. It was okay for the guys to go away together, but Myrna had heard the men gossip about women's conferences as "queers drinking beers."

Kelly had an easier time of it, working in her department for 15 years before coming out. She was attractive, vivacious, and friendly. Everyone knew she was close to her large family but no one ever asked her how her four days off went or who she was dating, which were common kitchen table topics among the guys. Sometimes a coworker asked her on a date, to which she always replied that she thought it was a bad idea to date someone she worked with. No one ever pressed the issue. While she often felt isolated, she was actually relieved to keep her private life private.

When a woman was appointed mayor, a group of gay women police officers and fire fighters arranged a private meeting with the new mayor to inquire about getting domestic partner benefits. They got more than they bargained for. In the course of conversation, the mayor asked if any of the women in the room felt in danger of losing their jobs because of their sexual orientation. Everyone raised her hand. The mayor was shocked and pledged on the spot that their jobs were safe. They were to come to her directly if they ever had a problem.

Kelly was ecstatic. This was the kind of affirmation she and the other women needed to feel comfortable. As luck would have it, her very next shift she was in the weight room working out when Carl, a fellow fire fighter, asked her if she was seeing anyone. She got off the treadmill and replied to Carl, "This is the first time in all these years anyone has asked me anything personal, so I'm going to tell you." Then she pulled out photos of her long-time partner, Debi, their house, their two children, their dog, and their parrot. "Oh my God," Carl replied, "you have a whole life and I didn't know a thing about it."

Being out was a lot easier than Kelly thought, possibly because she was competent and well liked to begin with. And there were a lot of benefits. When Debi brought their children to the firehouse everyone fussed over them like they did over everyone else's children. Kelly sensed that the men admired her ability to be a mom and a fire fighter. And the straight women, some of whom had seemed wary around her, were friendlier and eager to trade stories about their kids. This was a welcome surprise. By coming out Kelly increased the number of things she had in common with her coworkers. She could be herself. It was a relief to sit around the coffee table and talk openly about her home life. Introducing her work family to her real family increased the size of her support system and deepened the friendships she already had.

Things are changing, but more slowly for women than for ethnic minorities. The New York City Fire Department has only 27 women on a force of 11,000. But in Minneapolis, Minnesota; Madison, Wisconsin; San Francisco, California; Boulder, Colorado; and Miami Dade County, Florida, women account for 13–16% of the force. The California Department of Forestry is the largest single employer of women fire fighters, with 229 in a force of 3,412. More than 900 departments employ women fire fighters and very few major departments have yet to hire their first woman. The first generation of career women fire fighters is coming of age and the number of career fire service women at the chief officer level and beyond increases every year. Numbers are harder to capture in the volunteer service, but where they are tracked, the percentage of women seems to be on the rise.

Tips for Dealing with Diversity

- Choose your department carefully and do it as a family. This is the most important decision you'll make. What is the climate of the department? Is there administrative and supervisory support for women and minorities? For gays and lesbians? How committed is the department to fairness for everyone? Are there lawsuits pending based on race, gender, or sexual orientation issues? Is the workforce polarized around these issues? Do you see successful people who look like you? Being a pioneer creates extra stress on everyone, fire fighter and family alike.

(cont.)

(continued from previous page)

- Never push anyone to come out, speak up, file a lawsuit, or start a grievance. These are tough decisions and the person who must live with the consequences is in the best position to decide how to proceed.
- Know your rights. Stay up to date on what constitutes sexual harassment or discrimination. Learn about the differences between hazing and harassment based on race, sex, religion, or sexual orientation. Know what to do when your rights have been violated. See Resources for reading material and organizations that will help.
- Get a mentor to guide you, coach you, and kick you into gear. Women and minorities may be excluded from informal networks where a lot of learning takes place. Majority males will often not correct women or men of color for fear of being accused of harassment. Covering incompetence makes you a victim of social promotion. Anyone can be a mentor in the loose sense of the word: even bad managers can teach you something.
- Know your limits. Ask for help when you need it, but don't allow yourself to be protected or made a token. Either one will derail your learning, set you aside, and impede your career.
- Develop your own support systems. Sometimes people overreact when women or minorities get together, even though white men have being doing it for years. You may take a little heat, but you'll gain more than you lose.
- Women: don't try to be "one of the guys." If you do manage to gain acceptance this way, you may turn out to be someone you don't like. Endurance, flexibility, cardiovascular health, and the ability to manage stress are as important as big biceps to be an effective fire fighter. You may have to add some "male" skills to your tool kit, but you don't have to relinquish or exchange who you are to do so.
- Fight stereotypes. Females should not let anyone assume that they don't want to be considered for certain jobs or for promotion because they are women, wives, or mothers.
- Have a bottom line. Let people know what subjects are off-

limits for you. Enjoy humor, but don't put up with jokes that are demeaning or insulting to yourself or others. When someone violates your bottom line, confront that person in private, in a calm and firm way.

- The fire service is a paramilitary organization. Many women who haven't served in the military or played team sports can overreact to being yelled at. Prepare yourself.

- Avoid being drawn into conversation about or criticism of other women or minorities. Be careful not to be harder on other women or men of color than you are on the white male majority.

- Learn your history. Many younger women and minority fire fighters complain about having to listen to stories about the "bad old days." Pioneers deserve your respect for paving the way. Conversely, if you're a veteran fire fighter, consider mentoring the new hires. Give them the benefit of your hard-won experience while giving them the space to have things easier.

- Women: learn about male psychology. One mother said that now that she has a son she understands men better and her life as a fire fighter would have been easier had she had children first.

- Keep your eye on the prize. When the going gets rough remember your efforts will sow benefits for others who come after you.

- If your fire fighter is a victim of harassment or discrimination, encourage him or her to get mental health counseling or peer support. Victims of harassment, particularly if they have insufficient support from their departments, often need help to manage depression or anxiety, particularly if they're involved in a grievance or lawsuit.

- Have a support system of your own. You may need someone to fortify you while you buoy up your mate, especially if you're a target of the same bias that affects your loved one.

- Be a confidence builder, problem solver, and listener. Argue with catastrophic thinking. People who have a "deal with it" attitude and the confidence to challenge sexist, racist, and

(cont.)

129

(continued from previous page)

homophobic attitudes seem to fare better than those who feel helpless or ashamed.

Majority Fire Fighters and Their Families

- Avoid jealousy by getting to know your mate's coworkers. Concentrate on the strengths and weaknesses of your own relationship before assuming the source of the trouble is someone else.
- Remind yourselves that it's normal to feel angry and frustrated when you feel as though you're being punished for long-standing social problems that you didn't create and that are beyond your control.
- Lost opportunities are bound to happen as our society struggles and experiments with multiculturalism and diversity. It helps to be prepared for the possibility that your career may be affected.
- Choose your battles well. Learn to separate behavior from intentions and intentions from consequences. We all say things we regret. Learn to apologize.
- Don't be quick to assume that your majority status is what keeps you from certain opportunities. You may be overlooking something about yourself that you can change to your advantage.
- Use the experience of being shut out to understand how much damage discrimination inflicts on everyone.
- Don't put all your eggs in the "fire fighter" basket. Find other ways besides work to feel valued and enjoy community.

CHAPTER 8

Injuries and Fatalities

Hope and fear are enduring features of the human
experience . . . it is unlikely that people are going
to abandon them anytime soon just because
some psychologist told them they should.
—JON GERTNER,
quoting psychologist Daniel Gilbert

Nearly every day fire fighters somewhere lift heavy, often combative, patients, perform intimate medical procedures on people who
are filthy or who may have serious communicable diseases, leap
from planes into raging forest fires, drag heavy equipment into
burning buildings, inhale toxic fumes, expose themselves to hazardous materials, stand in the middle of busy freeways trying to
extricate people trapped in cars, rescue victims from confined
spaces, stand in or near collapsing structures, walk across roofs,
maneuver large and small vehicles, drive to and from the job, handle heavy machinery, get jolted awake from a dead sleep, dash
outdoors in all kinds of weather, execute water rescues, and participate in training exercises and simulations. In between times,
they drink coffee, study, smoke cigarettes, work out in the gym,
make inspections, maintain equipment, perform clean-up duty,
give public presentations, watch TV, and try to eat their meals in
peace. And this is not an exhaustive list of labors.

So, given all the potentially lethal and nonlethal activities in
the fire service, how perilous is fire fighting compared to other
professions? This question concerns every family. Whether or not

they say it aloud, families worry about fire fighter safety. Being told not to worry doesn't help and may even be insulting. What does seem to help is accurate information placed in proper perspective. The facts and figures in this chapter don't make for easy reading, but they are a lot more reliable—and maybe even comforting—than getting information from TV, movies, war stories, or your own untested worst fears.

INJURIES

Injuries are a fact of fire fighter life. In 2002, approximately 80,800 fire fighters were injured in the line of duty. This sounds like a large number, and it is, but it represents *all* types of injuries, not just those on the fireground. Actually, this number is the lowest reported since 1977 when the National Fire Protection Administration (NFPA) started collecting information from nearly 3,000 departments. About 14,600 of these injuries resulted in lost time, meaning they were serious enough to take the fire fighter off work.

Fifty percent of all the injuries reported occurred while fighting fires, which is consistent with statistics kept for other years. Most of these injuries were caused by overexertion or by falling, slipping, or jumping. The types of injuries reported included strains, sprains, muscular pain, wounds, cuts, bleeding, bruising, burns, and smoke or gas inhalation.

Regionally, the densely populated Northeast had the highest fireground injury rate, almost twice the rate for the rest of the country. The larger the population a department protects, the more fires there are to respond to and the higher the risk for injury. Fire fighters protecting communities of a quarter- to a half-million people carry 10 times the risk of getting hurt on the fireground because they respond to 240 times as many fires as do fire fighters working in departments that protect communities of less than 2,500.

About 15,000 injuries happened on duty but off the fireground during activities such as inspections and maintenance. A nearly equal number occurred at nonfire emergencies such as rescues, hazardous material calls, and natural disasters. About 5,800 injuries happened while responding to or returning from calls, and nearly 7,000 took place during training.

Strains, sprains, and muscular pain accounted for more than half of all nonfireground injuries. Rescue and EMS work are ergonomically very challenging. Both involve lifting heavy objects, twisting, making sudden movements, stretching, reaching, crawling in confined spaces, working when tired, driving over bumpy roads, and bouncing around in the back of an ambulance.

Invisible Injuries

There are a lot of numbers in this chapter about when, where, and how fire fighters get injured. But numbers don't tell the whole story. There is an emotional side to physical injury that is nearly invisible to all but the injured person and his or her family. Normally active and healthy people, especially professional rescuers, don't make good patients. They can be filled with anguish, anger, fear, and impatience about their condition. They put up a brave front for their friends, but their family gets the fallout.

Bud was strong and athletic before he was caught in a building collapse during a structure fire. He sustained multiple injuries to his shoulders, back, and neck. His injuries were not life threatening but they did threaten his career. The doctors told him to be patient, it would take time to heal. His family told him to be patient, they didn't want him rushing back to work and reinjuring himself.

Bud was 37 but felt like his 85-year-old grandfather. It was humiliating letting his wife, Deb, help him with intimate functions like bathing and going to the bathroom. Fire fighter friends helped around the house and drove Bud to physical therapy, but he still felt badly knowing how big a load Deb had to carry by herself.

When he got better Bud started dropping in at the firehouse. Both he and Deb thought that would cheer him up, but they were wrong. He was hurt when the guys joked about laying around and collecting disability pay. Even more alarming were sudden episodes of emotion when he would find himself fighting back tears because he couldn't bear not being part of the action. He stopped dropping by—it was easier not to see what he was missing.

At home he barked at Deb and the kids. Deb barked back; she had run out of patience with Bud's moods. Finally the department psychologist recommended that Bud be evaluated for antidepressants and arranged for him to attend a support group for people with chronic pain. The psychologist also worked with the whole family for a few sessions and helped them talk about how they were coping individually and as a family with the impact of Bud's injuries and uncertain future.

When Bud returned to modified duty, he was glad to have something useful to do. As much as he longed to go back on full duty, the closer the date, the more anxious he became. He worried that the men he had worked with preferred his replacement. He was certain everyone was watching to see if he was truly up to the job. If he got hurt again he didn't think he could survive another long rehabilitation. His psychologist told him such concerns were normal, to which Bud responded, "Not for me, Doc." One thing he knew for sure: he would never again joke about injured fire fighters milking the system or ignore their invisible injuries.

EXPOSURES

The NFPA has recently begun separately tracking exposures to hazardous and toxic materials along with diseases, rather than lumping them in with injuries. (Separating exposures statistically partly accounts for the reported long-term decrease in injuries.) Studies estimate that in 2001 there were 12,500 exposures to infectious diseases such as hepatitis, meningitis, HIV, TB, and so on. This is the equivalent of one exposure per 1,000 emergency medical runs. There were an estimated 20,000 exposures to hazardous materials like asbestos, radioactive substances, chemicals, and fumes, the equivalent of about 20 exposures per 1,000 hazardous condition runs.

Exposure to communicable diseases varies depending upon the population served. It's common sense; the risk is lower in areas where the population has a low rate of infectious disease. The risk of HIV infection in EMS workers following a needle stick— the most common cause of transmission—is very small. During a

45-year work life, there will be 180 cases of infection for every 100,000 workers.

Despite myths to the contrary, studies of thousands of fire fighter/paramedics over a nine-year period conclude that they are not at greater risk of infection from hepatitis C than the general population. The most important risk factors for getting hepatitis C are behavioral, not occupational: a history of blood transfusions, sexually transmitted diseases, and so on. The incidence of hepatitis B infection among health workers and fire fighters, while higher than the general population, has been substantially reduced since a vaccine became available. (The vaccine is less immediately effective for fire fighters who smoke or are obese.)

On the positive side, half of all paid fire departments in the United States conform to the Centers for Disease Control and Prevention (CDC) and the Occupational Safety and Health Administration (OSHA) standards. The rest, paid and volunteer alike, are covered by state laws that must be at least as strict as those of the federal OSHA. NFPA and OSHA have developed a number of ways to reduce the risk of exposure and contamination: proper disposal of needles; decontamination and disposal of contaminated waste and equipment; the use of personal protective equipment such as gloves, gowns, face shields, and ventilation devices; safety training and education; vaccinations; maintenance of confidential health files; postexposure evaluations; and infection control measures in the design of fire station bathrooms, kitchens, sleeping areas, and laundry facilities. One two-year study of fire fighter/EMT personnel reported a 51% decrease in the number of reported blood-borne pathogen exposures. The study attributed this decline to employee education.

BELLS AND WHISTLES

It used to be that everyone in the firehouse would wake up to clanging bells when there was an emergency in the middle of the night. It's a real shock to the system to go from a dead sleep to a dead run. The alarm itself, separate from the exertion of fire fighting, raises the responder's heart rate within 30 seconds, creates surges of adrenaline, and increases production of stress-related chemicals.

That's the rhythm of an emergency responder's life: long periods of inactivity punctuated by unpredictable periods of peak physical and psychological effort. The active periods are announced by beepers, bells, whistles, lights, sirens, blasts on the fire horn, or tones over a radio. Fire fighters, paramedics, and EMTs, whether volunteer or paid, may be the only people, besides the military, who must respond to a potentially life-threatening emergency from a state of sleep. It doesn't make any difference if it turns out to be a false alarm—as many do—your body has already revved up for an emergency.

Studies indicate that these sudden spurts of intense strenuous activity are implicated in cardiovascular illness, especially heart attacks. What's more, exertion, stress, and fatigue have all been shown to impair one's ability to think straight. This is especially true during fireground operations, where heat stress, danger, and extreme activity such as climbing ladders and dragging hose line push the active fire fighter to maximal heart rates. This is also true for EMS responders.

While it is impossible to eliminate emergency calls, the good news is that positive steps have been taken to minimize the stress involved. Many fire departments have modernized and civilized their "ring down" procedures. No longer is everyone one jolted awake by clanging bells, whether it's their call or not.

SLEEP DEPRIVATION

If you ski, you know how often skiers get hurt on the last run of the day, when they're tired. But skiers have the option to quit before they're exhausted, emergency responders do not. Fire fighters rarely sleep well. They're certain that the minute they fall deeply asleep they'll get a call. Some never allow themselves anything more than a restless catnap. When a call does come in, it is often difficult to go back to sleep. When you are abruptly awakened, particularly between the hours of 4:00 and 9:00 A.M., when you should be slumbering deeply, there's a consequence to pay in terms of fatigue, loss of concentration, impaired reaction time, irritability, and fuzzy thinking. Running on empty is risky.

Families may underestimate the toll fatigue and sleep deprivation takes. Over the years, I've heard fire fighters complain that their families think they lounge on the job, catching naps in their recliners. It depends on the department, but in some places a fire fighter can be called out 14 times in one 24-hour shift and end up with less than one hour's sleep. Even in slow houses fire fighters have lots to do between calls: inspections, equipment maintenance, household chores, training, studying, and so on. If families don't know this, I can only conclude it's because their fire fighters didn't tell them and/or their departments don't offer family orientations.

Unfortunately, humans can't "bank" sleep or easily make up for lost sleep. This is particularly true for night-shift workers and those who rotate shifts. Shift work is the equivalent of chronic jet lag. That grumpy, muddle-headed person who comes home from work or a call probably isn't lazy, or even in a bad mood; he or she may be suffering from exhaustion or sleep deprivation.

INJURIES OF THE FUTURE?:
HOMELAND PROTECTION AND BIOTERRORISM

"Sniff and get stiff" is a fire fighter's way of making light of a heavy subject. It describes what may happen in case of a chemical spill or gas attack. Since 9/11 all public safety workers and their families have unthinkable new worries. You know for certain that in the event of a terrorist attack, your fire fighter will be running toward the incident, away from you and away from safety.

None of us has a crystal ball. It may be wisest to follow the old adage: hope for the best and prepare for the worst. Feeling helpless just leads to anxiety. It is far better to get busy and do something constructive. I live in earthquake country and I keep a box of supplies in my car in case I get stranded. I have a blanket, toilet paper, water, food, a flashlight, a first aid kit, something to read, and an extra pair of glasses. I know full well that if an overpass collapses on my car, I'll have little use for my emergency supplies, but I feel better for having made these preparations and maybe they will come in handy in some other disaster.

All over the United States, at local, state, and federal levels, people are strategizing about homeland security. The first order of business is to prevent future attacks. Second on the list—and it's a close second—is to protect our emergency responders and health care workers, so that they can protect the rest of us. There are a lot of brave, bright people working hard on this problem.

FATALITIES

In 1997, the U.S. Bureau of Labor reported that fire fighters were three times more likely to be killed on the job than all other workers, but *ninth* on an index of relative risk. That means it's nine times riskier to be a logger or to fish professionally; eight times more risky to pilot an aircraft; and twice as risky to work in construction, drive a truck, be a roofer, or be a farmer. These comparisons are based on the number of hours fire fighters actually fight fire, perhaps two hours a month in some places, and the number of hours a logger logs or a truck driver drives. When you look at it this way, the risk factors change. Fire fighting itself can be exceptionally dangerous. But keep in mind that 80% of all fire service calls are medical.

In 2000, the numbers were lower: fire fighters were not even in the top 15 occupations at risk of fatal injury. Their risk was slightly more than twice that of the average worker, an improvement of nearly 46% since the 1997 data. Then came 2001 and the World Trade Center tragedy. Three hundred and forty fire fighters died in this one event, more than died in structure fires over the previous 11 years, counting both career and volunteer personnel. And more than died over the previous 20 years counting only full-time career fire fighters! Compare these figures to the 99 fire fighter fatalities that occurred in all other on-duty circumstances throughout the United States in 2001, a figure that has remained relatively steady for two decades. Unfortunately, recently released statistics show a disturbing upward trend: there were 102 on-duty fatalities in 2002 and 110 in 2003.

The loss of even one fire fighter is one too many. Still, it's important to remember that these fatalities are but a fraction of the million-plus career and volunteer fire fighters who work in the U.S. fire service.

These figures are collected by the NFPA, an international nonprofit membership organization founded in 1896. Every year since 1977, the NFPA has collected data about on-duty fire fighter fatalities in the United States. Their statistics include career and volunteer departments, seasonal and full-time employees of state and federal fire suppression agencies, prison inmates serving on fire-fighting crews, military personnel involved in fire fighting, civilian fire fighters working at military installations, and members of industrial fire brigades.

The good news is that the incidence of fatalities decreased from a high of 171 in 1978 to a low of 77 in 1992. The bad news is that it has since begun to inch upward. The puzzling news is that, while there has been a decline in fire incidents since 1983, the rate of fire fighter fatalities per 100,000 incidents has risen 25%.

From 1990 to 2000, the leading cause of fatal injuries was heart attacks. Fire fighters as a group are more likely than other U.S. workers to die of heart attacks while on duty. This statistic has remained constant for the past 16 years. Family reports and autopsies show the most common preexisting conditions for heart attack deaths are arteriosclerosis (the progressive hardening of the arteries), followed by prior heart attacks and hypertension. (Wildland fire fighters, who account for 8% of all fatalities, are an exception. They are more likely to be killed by traumatic injuries, and significantly less likely to die of heart attacks. This is because they are required to meet exceptionally high standards of physical fitness and they are considerably younger than their other fire service colleagues: nearly 70% of all part-time wildland fire fighters are under age 30.)

Trauma, including internal injuries and head injuries, was the second leading cause of death, followed by asphyxiation and burns. Most fatalities (67%) occurred at structure fires or wildland fires, and the majority of victims (60%) were front-line fire fighters.

Fire fighters of all ages were likely to have been engaged in emergency duties at the time of their deaths; most were fighting fires, many were responding to the scene, and some were engaged in suppression support. Emergency medical services (EMS) accounted for only 3% of the fatalities, with most of these resulting from collisions while transporting patients. One percent of fatalities occurred while fire fighters were engaged in physical fitness activities. Seven percent died while in training, usually from a heart attack. The dangers of live-fire exercises are well known and well publicized, so you may be surprised to learn that live-fire exercises are less lethal than equipment/apparatus drills.

The risk of fatal injury is markedly different for the paid and volunteer services. Nationally, almost three-quarters of all fire departments are staffed by volunteers, 21% are combination volunteer and career, and 6% are all career. Numerically speaking, the majority of deaths (57%) were volunteer fire fighters. However, paid personnel, who comprise about one-fourth of the total fire service workforce, were killed at a rate disproportionate to their numbers. (The likely reason for this is that career departments protect about 85% of the population and subsequently have a higher call volume.)

Why are volunteer fire fighters more at risk? There seems to be two major factors: age and vehicle accidents. About 40% of volunteer fire fighters are over 50 years old, compared to only 25% of the career service. About 60% of those who died on duty were over the age of 40. Younger fire fighters, age 35 or less, are more likely to be killed by traumatic injury than to die of a heart attack or stroke. After age 35, the proportion of deaths due to medical causes rises.

Since 1984, motor vehicle accidents have accounted for nearly one-quarter of all fire fighter deaths. About 25% of these deaths occurred in the fire fighter's own car. A significant majority of those who died were volunteers responding to a call from home or work. Accidents that involved department apparatus were most often associated with tankers transporting water in rural areas that lack local water sources. (Tankers are notoriously unstable and difficult to control due to water shifting in the tank.) Rural areas are almost exclusively protected by volunteer personnel. Remarkably, only 21% of the fire fighters who were killed in these accidents were wearing their seat belts!

Arson is the number-one killer of fire fighters in fire-related incidents. Since the arsonist's objective is to destroy, these fires can burn quickly and go undetected for a long time. By the time they are reported, they may be fully engaged and dangerous.

Where you live is also a risk factor. For example, Britain and Japan have fewer fire fighter fatalities than the United States, a phenomenon often explained by differences in their rules of engagement and guidelines for determining acceptable risk. In the United States, fatalities in structure fires are more common in the densely populated East, and wildland fire fatalities are more common in the West. You might think that states with high populations would have more fire fighter deaths, but this is not uniformly true. For example, New York and Pennsylvania have many more fire fighter fatalities than California and Texas, even though California and Texas have larger populations. The populations of New York and Texas are nearly comparable, yet New York has more than twice as many fire fighter fatalities as Texas. Population alone doesn't explain these differences. Experts suggest that more research is needed on the effect of variations in climate, types of housing, fire fighter safety codes, fire fighter age, types and frequencies of calls (structure fires, wildland fires, EMS), building code regulations, and the ratio of career to volunteer personnel.

HELP FOR GRIEVING FAMILIES

Should you or someone you know have the misfortune to lose a loved one in the line of duty, you will have support and plenty of it. Aside from family and friends, your department or your local area may have a fire chaplain, a staff psychologist, an employee assistance program, or a peer support team. One of the most helpful support systems will be the National Fallen Firefighters Foundation (NFFF). The NFFF is a tax-exempt, nonprofit organization created by Congress in 1992. Its purpose is to honor the memory of fallen fire fighters and provide support and assistance to surviving families and coworkers.

The NFFF Fire Service Survivors Network is composed of survivors who volunteer to reach out to each other and to the newly bereaved. The foundation tries to match people facing similar experiences and circumstances—for example, women who were pregnant when their husbands were killed, parents who lost children, and children who lost parents. Each October, the NFFF sponsors a Memorial Weekend on the National Emergency Training Center campus at Emmitsburg, Maryland. Families and departments of fire fighters being honored are invited to attend, and members of the Survivors Network return to greet new families and participate in the weekend's activities.

The NFFF also offers a variety of grief brochures for surviving families, friends, and coworkers. (A list of brochures is on their information-packed website along with information about their programs and about survivor benefits. Brochures may be ordered online. See Resources.) The foundation has a lending library of books, audiotapes, and videotapes, and publishes a quarterly newsletter for survivors that focuses on family issues, provides information on benefits and programs, and helps survivors stay in touch with each other.

We are all going to die sooner or later, on or off the job. Nothing complicates and intensifies grief more than discovering that your loved one has left no provisions or directions for her survivors, or worse, left everything to his first wife. It is an act of kindness and responsibility to have clear directives about end-of-life issues, both medical and financial. Even though it's hard to contemplate dying, don't postpone drafting a will, arranging for medical power of attorney, and making your wishes known.

Rico's department required that each employee fill out a form to be used in the event of a line-of-duty death. This form was part of a binder given to the family. The binder included worksheets and logs to record information: the location of important papers, insurance forms, bank account numbers, and so on; plans for the family to communicate through out-of-state relatives should the phone system go down; telephone numbers for the children's babysitters and names of the schools they attend. A copy of Rico's line-of-duty death form was kept under lock and key at the fire department.

When Rico died on the job, his department knew Rico wanted to notify his family and also knew that his parents were in poor health and didn't speak English. Instead of sending the fire chief, whom Rico disliked, to make the notification, the department sent one of his shift-mates who was a close friend. The department sent his captain, who spoke Spanish, to his parents' home; he was accompanied by paramedics, just in case either parent had a medical crisis in response to the terrible news. Rico also left very clear directions about the circumstances under which he wanted his doctors to keep him alive. His will indicated that he wanted to be cremated and not buried, which saved his wife from having a painful argument with his parents, who were opposed to cremation and wanted Rico buried in the family plot.

Tips for Protecting Your Fire Fighter and Yourself

- Encourage your loved one to eat a healthy diet, exercise regularly, maintain a reasonable weight, stop smoking, and consume alcohol in moderation. If you can't get your fire fighter to cooperate, model a healthy lifestyle yourself. A new study of 4,700 couples showed that there is a strong association between the health of husbands and the health of wives. Married people tend to follow the same kinds of diets, for better or worse, or to smoke if their spouse does.
- Encourage your entire family to get regular physical examinations and to pay attention to doctor's advice.
- Never give up, because it's never too late. Stan and Edna are in their fifties. They walk in the hills near their home several times a week, and go to the local gym to lift weights and take a weekly yoga class. Stan wouldn't have been caught dead in a gym and he thought yoga was for weirdoes until Edna signed them up for a year, and had the monthly dues automatically paid by credit card. At 58 dollars a month, that was less than a dollar a day for each of them. Stan hates to pay for something he doesn't use and he doesn't like being alone, so he went along muttering under his breath. Guess what? The benefits of both, weight lifting especially, were so pronounced and so rapid, that Stan never misses a session, even when Edna can't go.
- Encourage your department to create a wellness program that includes families (see Chapter 9 for more information).

(cont.)

(continued from previous page)

- Buckle up your seat belt and encourage your fire fighter to do the same, every time he or she gets in a vehicle. (Fire fighters who buckle up at home often don't take the same precautions at work because they are rushing or wearing equipment that makes buckling up awkward.) Saving a few seconds is not worth risking your life.
- Make certain your own home is fire-safe and that you have installed smoke alarms, or, better still, a sprinkler system. It is ironic how few fire fighters practice what they preach. Sprinkler systems save lives and money: some insurance companies will reduce their premiums when you install a system and many communities now require them in new homes.
- Volunteer to start a program or help out with an existing program that educates the public, both adults and children, about fire safety. The fewer fires there are, the lower the risk that your fire fighter will be killed or hurt on the job.
- Start a spousal support network in your department and/or join an existing one. Team up with others to provide emotional and practical support to the families of fire fighters who are ill, injured, or have been killed. It will help them feel less isolated and overwhelmed and help you feel more in control.
- Departments should have a systematic way of maintaining contact with sick or injured fire fighters who are out on long-term disability rather than counting on family to shoulder the entire load. Consider encouraging your department to start a peer support team or a buddy system for disabled fire fighters.

CHAPTER 9

Fitness, Health, and Safety

Somebody once suggested to me that psychologists were naive because we thought that if we could explain something we would cure it. It was an interesting observation with a kernel of truth in it. I know that describing or explaining the improvements made in fitness, health, and safety won't end fire fighter family concerns. But I believe that learning about these advances, technological and otherwise, will broaden your perspective and ease your worries. An enormous amount of energy and thought is being expended on safety by all sectors of the fire service—labor and management—and by several federal agencies dedicated to worker safety.

HEALTH AND FITNESS

Fire fighters are braver and tougher than many of the rest of us. But they are just as susceptible to overeating and underexercising. One of my colleagues (who would not want his name to be used) told me that he thought the most dangerous thing a fire fighter did was eat lunch! On one of my visits to the Midwest, I spent several days living in a fire station. Though I was assured it was not the norm, four out of the five days all three shifts ate their lunch and dinner at fast-food restaurants. The favorite breakfast food was doughnuts from the vending machine. Snacks came from an unending stream of home-baked goodies delivered by well-meaning friends and family who just wanted a reason to drop in and visit.

Of course, there are no guarantees. Being fit or not smoking doesn't ensure that you won't have a heart attack, but both reduce the risk. And fitness makes sense in dollars and cents. For example, it costs approximately $88,000 to hire and train a fire fighter, $500 per day in overtime to fill in for an injured worker, and about $450,000 for a fire fighter's premature retirement. The Seattle Fire Department, which employs about 1,100 fire fighters, spends nearly 2.6 million dollars a year in disability costs. The department's total budget is 98 million dollars.

The fire service itself has recognized the need to improve the overall fitness of its workers. In 1997, the IAFF and the IAFC drafted the Fire Service Joint Labor Management Wellness/Fitness Initiative, a program designed for incumbent fire service personnel. It incorporates a fitness evaluation (strength, flexibility, and cardiovascular health), a medical evaluation (including evaluation of vision, hearing, and respiratory function; chest x-rays; tests for diabetes, TB, and hepatitis C; vaccination for hepatitis B; etc.), and a rehabilitation component—often run by fire fighters who have been specially trained and certified—for those who need it. Behavioral health information and assistance in weight reduction, smoking cessation, stress management, and nutrition are also important parts of the initiative, as is systematic data collection. So far, the databank consists of 35,000 fire fighters.

These days most career departments allow crews one hour per shift for physical training. Many have added workout rooms into their station designs and routinely budget for new or replacement fitness equipment. Volunteers may not be so lucky. An estimated 792,000 fire fighters, most of them volunteers serving small communities, work in departments with no programs for maintaining basic fire fighter fitness and health.

Why doesn't every fire department in the country embrace the fitness initiative? The reasons are different in different places. Career fire fighters sometimes worry that such programs are a way for management to terminate unfit fire fighters and they are also concerned about confidentiality. They fear that management, always mindful of money, may find it easier to blame individual fire fighters than to bankroll long-term fitness programs. On the other hand, labor may attribute health problems, such as muscular strains, to the work environment (poorly designed equipment, insufficient staffing, etc.) and downplay personal factors such as fitness. Who's right? We don't really know. Who's caught in the middle? The fire fighter and his or her family.

There is another angle to consider. Fitness and job-relevant performance standards are not the same. Out-of-shape or aging incumbent fire fighters are frequently able to pass performance tests. If they can't, there will be consequences—consequences that one hopes are delivered in supportive, not intrusive or punitive, ways. This is an extremely sensitive and emotional issue because it tends to affect aging fire fighters who may be legends in their departments and held in high esteem by their colleagues.

I had arranged to interview Milt and his wife, Donna, in their spacious suburban home. It was the holiday season and their house was decorated for Christmas inside and out. School was on vacation and their teenage daughter, Angie, a tall, athletic-looking, young woman, was at home, so we invited her to join our discussion. Her father works in a large urban department that has recently hired a lot of women. I asked her if she was interested in following in her father's footsteps. She responded immediately, "Women don't belong in the fire service—they aren't strong enough do the job." Her mother and father nodded their heads in agreement.

I asked her father if he wouldn't rather depend on a young fit female to rescue him in a crisis than one of the middle-aged, overweight, cigarette smokers I'd met in his department. Dad was adamant: he trusted the fat fire fighter to have the courage, the "heart," and the experience to function in an emergency. He didn't know what these young women were capable of doing and he couldn't count on them. "I grew up with these guys," he said. "I knew them when they were in good shape." Milt may be old-fashioned and behind the times, but I couldn't help thinking how lucky people are to have friends and family who remember them this fondly as they grow old.

How Fit Is Fit?

This is an arguable point. No one is suggesting that fire fighters be held to a level of athletic fitness, but they must be able to perform the job. With your doctor's permission, put yourself to this test designed by Lieutenant Michael Cacciola of the Fire Department of New York City's Fire Academy and see how you do.

1. Simulated stair climbing: walk on a stair climber at a rate of 59 steps per minute for five minutes, 12 seconds. If you stop or grab onto the handrails, you fail.
2. Simulated hose advance: fill a wheelbarrow with 70 pounds of rocks, grab the handles backward, so you're facing away from it, and then walk forward, moving the wheelbarrow 90 feet in 46 seconds.
3. Simulated rescue of an unconscious victim: fill a wheelbarrow with 130 pounds of rocks, grab the handles so that you're facing it, then walk backward 55 feet in 24 seconds.
4. Simulated ceiling pulldown: Press two 30-pound dumbbells over your head three times. Then weight a lat-pulldown machine with 80 lbs. and pull it to your waist five times. Repeat this sequence for 60 seconds, rest for 30 seconds, then repeat again. You'll need a total of 20 repetitions in four sets to pass, or, as the author warns, "pass out."

A Model Fitness Program for Fire Fighters

Health professionals generally agree on a multipronged approach to health and fitness. In an ideal world, this is the kind of program all fire fighters should follow. Many of the components are easily adapted for families, suggesting that department-sponsored fitness programs could and perhaps should be extended to family members. The results might just be increased motivation and consistency.

1. *Do strength-training and flexibility exercises.* Musculo-skeletal injuries account for almost half of all line-of-duty injuries. Regular strength training (weight lifting) and flexibility exercises

(stretching, yoga) have been shown to reduce the frequency of back injuries among fire fighters.

2. *Improve cardiovascular health.* As you now know, heart attacks are the number-one killer of fire fighters. While sudden intense bursts of strenuous or stressful activity pushes your cardiovascular system to its limit, being sedentary is the real risk factor. Regular, moderate cardiovascular workouts can improve cardiovascular health and make a significant contribution to weight control, which in turn helps lower blood pressure, reduce cholesterol, and decrease the risk of diabetes. High blood pressure, high cholesterol, diabetes, and poor aerobic capacity are all implicated in heart disease.

3. *Have regular physical checkups.* The NFPA recommends medical exams every three years for fire fighters who are younger than thirty, every two years for those in their thirties, and annually for those forty and older. Regular medical checkups can spot subclinical, nonsymptomatic warning signs of heart disease, diabetes, high blood pressure, respiratory disease, and some cancers. Some studies of fire fighter deaths suggest that there is more evidence that fire fighters are at risk for chronic heart disease than for any specific sudden-death events such as aortic aneurysm or heart attack.

Annual checkups should also include an assessment of hearing problems. Hearing loss is common in the fire service because of sirens, air horns, diesel engines, mechanized equipment, noisy fire stations, and the like.

4. *Stop smoking and chewing tobacco.* Fire fighters seem to smoke as much as the general population. But because studies show that fire fighters are routinely exposed to toxic materials and the products of combustion, smoking makes things worse for them. It amplifies respiratory problems, increases the frequency of respiratory symptoms, and is correlated with lung and heart disease. Smoking is one of the hardest habits to break. Some departments won't even hire people who smoke or chew tobacco. Check with your employee assistance program or local public health department for smoking cessation programs.

5. *Practice good nutrition.* Eat mindfully and healthily: enough, but not too much. If you're a friend or a family member, don't make food your ticket to the firehouse. Resist the TV ads:

there are many ways to show your love beside feeding people. If you want to visit, just visit. Bring flowers, not food. If you must, bring some healthy, low-calorie/low-fat treats.

6. *Drink less.* Use alcohol moderately. Find additional ways to relax and be sociable (see Chapter 12).

7. *Buckle up!* Use your seat belt at work and at home.

SAFETY

It used to be that the occupational perils facing fire fighters—acute and chronic health hazards; traumatic injuries; burns; smoke inhalation; damage to eyesight, hearing, and sense of smell; infectious diseases; cardiovascular problems; respiratory problems; nonmalignant respiratory disease; musculoskeletal injuries; some cancers; reproductive risks; and so on—were considered uncontrollable. This was the price fire fighters paid for having chosen a dangerous, public-service occupation that offered security, fun, and a lot of time off. That reasoning is no longer acceptable. Society needs fire fighters and recognizes, particularly after 9/11, the risks they take.

Over the past several decades, with more than a little shove from fire fighters themselves by way of their labor organizations, there has been increased attention to fire fighters' health and safety needs. While they may not always agree on how or when to do this, how bad the problem is, or what causes it, all the organizations listed below are pushing to eliminate the unnecessary hazards of fire fighting and to reduce the necessary ones: the International Association of Fire Fighters (IAFF), representing most career fire fighters; the National Volunteer Fire fighter Council (NVFC), representing most volunteers; the International Association of Fire Chiefs (IAFC); the National Fire Protection Association (NFPA); the International Fire Service Training Association (IFSTA); the National Association of Search and Rescue (NASAR); federal agencies that set standards for occupational health and safety like the National Institute for Occupational Safety and Health (NIOSH), the Occupational Safety and Health Administration (OSHA), the Centers for Disease

Control and Prevention (CDC); and many more I haven't mentioned.

Changes in the Firehouse

I am being given a tour of a brand-new fire station that is still under construction. It has soaring ceilings and tinted green windows. The kitchen is huge and beautifully equipped with a restaurant-style stove, two high-tech dishwashers, and gleaming stainless-steel counters. The apparatus bay is enormous, with automatic doors at each end. The only connection this new fire station has to tradition are framed photos of the old station, glass cases displaying antique brass nozzles and bells, and the ubiquitous La-Z-Boy loungers lined up in the TV room, still covered in plastic sheeting.

To my surprise the sleeping area is divided into single rooms. This is a new trend in firehouse architecture, and this financially well-heeled district is one of the few to be able to afford such "luxurious" accommodations for its staff. Individual rooms mean that men and women will not have to bunk together or share a bathroom. Each fire fighter will have some privacy—a quiet place to retreat from the TV or the noisy banter in the kitchen, to unwind in peace, read, or just sleep without having to contend with other people's snoring or smells. It may also help stop the spread of colds and flu and other air-borne illnesses that can easily circulate through dormitory-style accommodations. It all looks very appealing, but the fire fighters who are giving me the tour are clearly worried that separate rooms are a threat to their camaraderie, a prelude to the breakdown of the traditional social structure.

I'm looking for the brass pole when I realize this is a one-story firehouse. The truth of the matter is that fire poles are only rarely used, and then usually by younger fire fighters. The brass pole is an icon of fire service tradition dating back to the days of horse-drawn fire wagons when fire fighters lived upstairs and dalmatians and horses lived below. I've listened to lots of complaints about the loss of tradition, but rarely has anyone complained about the brass pole falling into disuse. Instead, I've heard stories about compression fractures and broken legs from landing wrong or sleepy fire fighters who missed the pole entirely and took a free fall to the floor below.

Equipment

I'm walking through the exhibit hall for the annual convention of the International Association of Fire Chiefs (IAFC), two gigantic floors jammed with vendors selling all manner of equipment from the massive to the miniscule. I walk past mobile computerized command centers, gargantuan tankers, green and red fire trucks resplendent with airbrushed murals depicting the fire heroes of 9/11, and rescue vehicles that are essentially giant, rolling toolboxes. It's like walking through a herd of grazing dinosaurs. Turn the corner and I'm in the land of the tiny: books, helmets, badges, T-shirts, and souvenir gee-gaws to bring home to the family.

Fire fighters are dependent on their equipment for safe being, and their equipment gets better, but not lighter, all the time. Fully dressed fire fighters wear a minimum of 50 pounds of gear, and this can go much, much higher depending upon the type of incident to which they're responding. Add a flashlight (five pounds), a Halligan tool and a flat-head ax (15 pounds), and perhaps a high-rise pack (65 pounds), and you see why fire fighters need to be physically fit. All this new equipment, while essential to improve safety, weighs a lot, retains heat, and increases the energy burden on the wearer.

Clothing

The manufacture of personal protective equipment, the pants and jacket commonly known as "bunker" or "turnout gear," is regulated by the National Fire Protection Agency (NFPA). Bunker gear is designed to protect a fire fighter's skin from flame and from steam, which is the number-one cause of burns, and to keep the fire fighter as cool as possible. Personal protective equipment has four layers: a flame-proof outer shell made from high-tech, space-age material; a vapor barrier protecting against steam and water; a thermal liner-insulator that captures air and dissipates heat; and a breathable face cloth that absorbs sweat and cools the wearer. This is a far cry from the days of leather and rubber and thigh-high boots.

Bunker gear has recently been "accessorized," if I may use that term, with a knitted, heat-resistant hood worn under the helmet, because cheeks and ears (and wrists) are vulnerable to getting burned. Not everyone welcomes wearing a hood, especially seasoned fire fighters who may have worked for years without one.

Jack, a 17-year career veteran from an urban department, is not happy with this modern gear. While it may protect better, he says it weighs more, makes him hotter, and masks his ability to read the radiant heat from a fire. "My ears are like canaries. If my ears burn, I'm in trouble and need to get out. A blistered ear is better than a melted mask." There is a lot of support for Jack's resistance to change and for not compromising his independent judgment: one training manual I read advised fire fighters to determine how hot a building was by taking off their gloves, but, the instructions continued, "Don't tell anyone."

Breathing Apparatus

Fire fighters operating in toxic environments wear a self-contained breathing apparatus (SCBA), a 28-pound cylinder filled with compressed air. The air supply is activated with a valve that cannot be turned off by mistake. The tank locks onto a face mask, and a regulator controls airflow, providing air on demand. When the air in the cylinder is at 25% capacity, a warning alarm goes off and the regulator shakes the face mask. A remote gauge in the personal alert safety system (PASS) console, described below, continuously shows how much air is left, so that fire fighters may individually calculate how much air they need to get to an exit. Depending on where they are, 25% may not be enough. (Wildland fire fighters, who work and live in smoky environments for days and weeks, do not use SCBA equipment because they are cumbersome in the brush and provide only a short supply of air.)

The usual SCBA tank is designed to last 30 minutes, depending on the fire fighter's fitness level and level of exertion. In physically demanding situations, a fire fighter can deplete his or her tank in as little as 10–15 minutes. SCBA came on the scene in the

1970s, and has had a positive influence in reducing pulmonary disease and respiratory problems among fire fighters. SCBA gear has also been shown to reduce the number of lung injuries during salvage and overhaul operations. After a fire is over, the air is still smoky and filled with the toxic by-products of combustion.

SCBA equipment is constantly being refined. New technology continues to move toward the ideal of a fail-safe system: flashing dots inside the face mask that can warn fire fighters that their air is low in case they are unable to hear their low-air alarms; adding a tone to a vibrating alert to signal others that a colleague is running out of air; and intercom systems integrated into the SCBA to eliminate radio traffic and allow for clearer communications.

Locators

Another advance is the personal alert safety system (PASS) device that was developed in the 1980s. The PASS clips to the SCBA harness and emits a loud signal when manually activated or when it has not sensed motion for 30 seconds, thereby alerting other fire fighters that a colleague is in distress and helping them to locate that person. (It's an "in" joke that the PASS device has a second use: it identifies fire fighters who are standing around not working.) The system sensor in the PASS is located in such a way that it will go off no matter which way you fall, whether face down or on your back. The National Institute for Occupational Safety and Health (NIOSH) found multiple occasions when fire fighters failed to wear or activate their PASS devices, prompting SCBA manufacturers to begin integrating PASS devices into SCBA systems so that they will now turn on automatically when the air cylinder is activated.

Ropes, Tools, and Gadgets

Fire fighters may carry bailout ropes so they can slide or rappel out of a building if their exit is blocked. There is something called a "fallen fire fighter harness" that can be sewn into personal protective equipment to effect a rapid rescue. It eliminates the need to find a rope, remove a fire fighter's jacket during rescue to avoid snags, or retrieve an extrication device and then attach the fallen fire fighter to that device. The "best dressed" fire fighters will supplement their protective clothing with rope systems and light sticks, chemically activated, self-contained sources of light.

The list of available accessories is endless, far too long to cover here. There are hose-exit arrows, raised tactile surfaces attached to the hose line at regular intervals. A hose line is a lifeline. Fire fighters read hose couplings in order to know which way is out. The effectiveness of this technique is reduced by the thick gloves they wear as well as by zero visibility conditions. When multiple crews are working off a single engine, hose accountability markers can identify a distressed crew's hose line from outside, allowing the rapid intervention crew (RIC) to improve accuracy and response time for a rescue. And if they have an emergency transfill hose or RIC bag, they can quickly and efficiently supply air to a fallen fire fighter under the most adverse conditions.

The bottom line is that there is always a need for better equipment and always a supply to fill that need. What is not in limitless supply is money, particularly during periods of fiscal crisis for government. In fact, a recent needs assessment issued by the NFPA indicated that 32% of all fire stations are nearly 40 years old and 50% of all engines are 15 years old. The report concluded that there are not enough portable radios to go around and decried the fact that one-third of fire fighters per shift are not equipped with SCBA, nearly half don't have PASS devices, and about 57,000 lack personal protective clothing, mostly in small volunteer departments. One-third of what they do have is 10 years old. It will take more than a bake sale to handle these expenses.

Incident Command Systems

Equipment is critically important, but it is not sufficient for ensuring safety. Information and personnel management are key. Bad or missing information can kill. It killed Bill.

Bill's department arrived on scene within minutes of the alarm, but the wooden fourplex apartment was already fully involved. Like many emergencies, this one looked like organized pandemonium: flashing lights, sirens, fire trucks, police cars, TV reporters, fire buffs, and journalists spilling into the street. Neighbors were everywhere, wearing winter coats and boots over their nightclothes. One of them raced over to Bill, a 10-year veteran, and identified himself as one of the tenants. "There's an old lady in the upstairs unit," he yelled over the noise, "I don't see her, I don't think she got out." Bill charged into the building in full rescue mode. He came out empty-handed and returned again twice. On his third try, he fell through a floor. Eighteen other fire fighters went in to rescue him. When they found him, they discovered that his PASS system had never been turned on and his radio wasn't working. Bill died in the hospital three weeks later. The old lady was out of town, visiting relatives.

Two things went dreadfully wrong here. First, Bill was "freelancing," a term for fire fighters who act individually, not as part of a team. Second, his department had not yet implemented the formal strategy for managing information and organizing personnel known as the Incident Command System (ICS) or Incident Management System (IMS). In any call, simple or complex, routine or emergency, involving single or multiple jurisdictions, it is as important to control and deploy personnel in a safe and effective manner as it is to deploy equipment and put out fire.

Departments are increasingly using the IMS or ICS system, and in some states it is actually mandated. Why should you be interested in this? Because it protects fire fighters. One whole sector of the IMC/ICS system is dedicated to fire fighter safety. It is managed by a designated safety officer whose exclusive job is to evaluate the hazard to fire fighters, make a safety plan, account for the whereabouts of all personnel at regular intervals, and alter or stop an operation when it is jeopardizing personnel.

Scott was the safety officer at a large, late-night warehouse fire that was billowing black smoke in all directions. As safety officer, he had to restrain his own instincts to run into the building with his coworkers. For one thing he loves fighting fires and doesn't get to do it much anymore. For another, it was a dangerous situation and he wanted to be there for his company and to help rescue any trapped civilians, although at this point neither Scott nor anyone else knew for certain that there were people inside. ICS protocol required that Scott relocate around the corner, out of sight of the fire, so that he could focus on strategy and analyze the firegound based on real information, not his gut instinct. Being safety officer is a hard job that requires discipline and emotional toughness. Scott did it because he was there when Bill was fatally injured, and he believes to this day that his friend might still be alive and 18 other fire fighters might not have jeopardized their safety trying to rescue him had there been an ICS system in place.

Two-In/Two-Out

Two-in/two-out is the fire fighters' buddy system. It is a standard procedure endorsed by the the Occupational Safety and Health Administration (OSHA). What this means is that when fire fighters are inside an area immediately dangerous to life and health (this happens often enough that there is a recognizable abbreviation: IDLH), they must maintain verbal or visual contact with at least one other fire fighter. Moreover, a team of at least two other properly equipped and trained fire fighters must be stationed outside before any teams enter the IDLH area—no freelancing, no rogue operations.

Staying in touch with your buddy may be easier said than done under some circumstances. In recognition of this, most modern fire service departments, career and volunteer, train fire fighters in self-rescuing techniques, such as sliding down a charged hose line, or rappelling with a rope, to name a few. In some states, self-rescue is required training.

ACCEPTABLE RISK: THE RULES OF ENGAGEMENT

Modern fireground operations proceed under specific rules of engagement. Basically, the rules say:

- We will risk our lives a little to save savable property.
- We will risk our lives a lot to save savable lives.
- We will not risk our lives for property or lives already lost.
- No building or any kind of property is worth the life of a fire fighter.
- No risk to the safety of fire fighters is acceptable in situations where there is no possibility of saving lives or property.

These rules make sense, but in fact there is no national or international consensus about exactly what constitutes acceptable risk, savable property, or savable lives. The British and Japanese fire services are said to have the strictest standards about acceptable risk; in the United States, the East Coast fire services are reputed to define acceptable risk more broadly than their West Coast counterparts.

Some fire service professionals think improvements in protective gear and equipment have produced a false sense of security and altered the ratio of risk. They worry that this false sense of security prompts fire fighters to fight fire more aggressively and to penetrate buildings more deeply, despite increased hazard from new and cheaper forms of building construction.

Six fire fighters in Worcester, Massachusetts, died in 1999 fighting a fire that was begun by vagrants in an abandoned warehouse. More fire fighters might have died had the chief not stopped them from entering the building in search of their fallen companions.

Questions abound after such a tragedy. Was the loss of life justified? Should fire departments risk their safety trying to save derelict buildings that have been forsaken by their owners? Does the life of a homeless vagrant call for less risk than the life of a child or a doctor? How shall we make these decisions, and how do we live with the ones we make?

The rules of engagement are logical and tactical, designed to take the emotion out of an incident. It is harder, though, to take emotions out of fire fighters, especially when their adrenaline is running high. This is why training, supervision, and command structures are so important to safety. Fighting fires is such a rarity—about two in 10 calls for service in many places—that fire fighters may take chances just to be part of the excitement and the action. After all, competency in the fire service is measured by how many fires you have fought, how many lives you have saved, how many chances you have taken.

Most fire fighters train in burn towers or single-family residences. Think of how eager some fire fighters must be to try their skills in a flaming warehouse 10 times the size of a three-bedroom home. This is a situation calling for different air management strategies and "deep penetration" techniques. Large buildings are not forgiving when you run out of air or get lost, and you can't escape fast enough if the building starts to fall apart.

Fire fighters have to be trained to stay calm under pressure, when their brain and endocrine system are pumping chemicals into their bloodstreams, producing an adrenaline-powered "high"— a sense of aliveness, energy, vitality, and alertness that can become its own reward. This powerful, primitive, and involuntary reaction may be what people mean when they say that the fire service is addictive and "gets in the blood." It may also be what creates statistics when fire fighters leap into their cars on the way to a call and don't buckle their seat belts, when they don't wear their SCBA, when they think they can beat gravity or traffic, when they intentionally ignore their low air alarms, when they don't buckle up inside an ambulance, when they or their departments dispatch every medical run, urgent or routine, as if it's a life-saving emergency. Like it or not, adrenaline and machismo can be significant factors in line-of-duty deaths and injuries.

TRAINING

Fire fighting is a low-frequency, high-risk operation. There are simply not enough fires anymore to rely on on-the-job training. As fire fighting becomes more complex, the importance of training becomes more critical. Gone are the days of simplistic technology: "surround and drown," "put the wet on the red."

Training, to be useful, must simulate real situations, which of course makes standardized training difficult because of the many variations in firegrounds: high-rise dwellings, industrial complexes, single-family dwellings, forests, airports, and so on. Training must also be constantly updated to keep pace with new developments in society.

For example, recent trends in building construction, such as lightweight truss construction, wooden I-beams, thermal-pane windows, rolled and/or blown-in insulation, and chipboard are a boon to homebuilders and a bane to the fire service. Combined with modern furnishings and finishes, there is increased potential for rapid flashovers, building collapses, and the release of toxic fumes. Consider the challenges inherent in fighting a deep-seated fire in a four-story apartment building when you don't know the layout of the building and visibility is impaired. Consider the additional challenges if the bulk of your training has been in one-story single-family residences.

None of this takes into consideration the increase in hazardous material incidents and the specter of bioterrorism and weapons of mass destruction. Clearly these have generated the need for new training in the fire service.

Rescue Teams

By now, many career and volunteer departments are training rapid intervention teams or crews (RITs/RICs) according to federal standards issued by the NFPA. RICs are trained to stand by on the fireground and deploy immediately when fire fighters inside a building are in danger. Besides their specialized training, RICs carry extra SCBA gear, ropes, extrication tools, ladders, special hose lines, and—if their departments can afford one—a thermal imaging camera.

I am standing in the rain watching a RIC team go through a training simulation. They are rescuing a downed fire fighter from a deep, narrow concrete pit by tying ropes into specialty knots, looping these around the downed fire fighter's legs and arms, and then hoisting her to safety. The exercise is repeated with several variations, including ones in which the downed fire fighter is able to assist the rescuers and others in which she is totally unconscious.

The exercise is modeled in memory of the 1987 death of John Nance, a 51-year-old veteran Columbus, Ohio, fire fighter who fell through the floor of a four-story, 11,500-square-foot building. Under unbearable fire conditions, his rescuers tried repeatedly to haul him up, and actually were able to grab his hands, but couldn't lift him high enough. They then tried to pull him out with a rope, but he apparently couldn't hold on. Then they enlarged the hole and dropped a ladder down to him. Perhaps exhausted and confused by elevated levels of carbon monoxide, he inadvertently climbed up the wrong side, hit his head on the floor joists and fell again. His fellow fire fighters tried to climb down into the hole and drag him up, but were driven back by fire. Several more last-ditch efforts were made to reach him from the outside, but the building was soon engulfed in flames.

This is fire fighter folklore at it's best and saddest. Unlike other professions—medicine and law enforcement, for example— the fire service openly shares its pain and errors along with its victories. Fire fighting is a culture built on chronicles of experience that serve as the foundation for future training.

We move next to another rescue exercise called the "Denver Prop," which is dedicated to the memory of Engineer Mark Langvardt, a 16-year veteran who died in an arson fire in 1992. Engineer Langvardt became trapped in a small room crammed with office furniture. The only way out was a small window blocked by a metal security gate. Fire fighters could not gain the leverage needed to lift the unconscious Langvardt—who was in full gear and drenched with water—through the window four feet above him.

The "Denver Prop" simulation takes place inside a training tower. The "rescuers" are panting and grunting from the effort to lift the "downed" fire fighter through a small opening. How hard this must be in a real fire, surrounded by heat and noise and blackness, falling debris, arcing electrical wires, desperate emotions, and everywhere something to snag your turnouts and get hung up in your SCBA gear.

The final challenge of the day is the mask confidence exercise. It is the most accurately simulated exercise of the morning. The objective is for a crew to find their way out of a dark, confined space crammed with hazards and filled with artificial, breathable smoke. They are to leave no one behind. This is uncharted territory—no one but the trainer is familiar with the course.

The first obstacle is a wall of studs so narrowly spaced that all the participants remove their air cylinders to get through. Next, they feel their way around the wall until they pass through some downed wires without becoming entangled. As they move ahead, they hit a dead end and retreat until they find a crawl space through which they inch forward, pushing their air tanks before them, probing for hazards and holes in the floor.

I am able to watch the whole exercise because the team has a new "toy," a thermal imaging camera that sees through smoke and can locate the source of heat, all the while sending images to an aboveground TV monitor. The exercise takes nearly 20 minutes to complete. When the team emerges from their subterranean playground, they are high with excitement. I share their pleasure at successfully completing this challenging exercise. I am, once again, in awe of their courage.

It's been a very educational day for me and I think how wonderful it would be if families were invited to observe training days like this. I think they'd be very interested, although I wonder how willing fire fighters would be to show them the dangers and risks involved. On the other hand, wouldn't families be relieved to see how fire fighters train and learn? How they practice safety procedures? Wouldn't they be pleased to be included and feel, as I did, a mix of admiration and pride?

CHAPTER **10**

Trauma and Stress

> Expect trouble in your life, because it will catch up
> with you sooner or later. Nobody escapes it. Trouble
> does not mean you are stupid or bad or guilty of
> some wrongdoing, it simply means you are a member
> of the human race. Remember it is not what happens
> to you that counts, but how you handle it.
> —ANN LANDERS, quoted in her obituary
> in the *San Francisco Chronicle*, June 23, 2002

WHAT'S CHANGED AND WHAT HASN'T

Since I wrote *I Love a Cop: What Police Families Need to Know* in 1997 there has been a lot of controversy and change in the treatment of trauma. Mental health experts and trauma researchers have been debating about what works and what doesn't, about who needs help, why, and under what circumstances. It's actually one of the hottest topics in psychology and, depending upon whom you talk to, the arguments are far from settled.

What hasn't changed are the sights, sounds, smells, and sadness that accompany injury and death. And the fact that many fire fighters see more tragedy in a few months or a few years than the rest of us will see in our entire lifetimes: shootings, drownings, knifings, bombings, beatings, hangings, car wrecks, train wrecks, airplane crashes, falls, fires, electrocutions, overdoses, poisonings, suffocations, incinerations, heart attacks, seizures, chronic illness, sudden illness, workplace violence, school violence, domestic vio-

163

lence, gang violence, and all manner of disasters, natural and un-natural, accidental and intentional.

In 2002, public fire departments responded to more than 21 million calls: 12,903,000 medical aid calls, 1,687,500 fire calls, 2,116,000 false alarms, 888,500 mutual aid calls, 361,000 hazardous material calls, 603,500 hazardous condition calls, and 2,744,000 calls the National Fire Protection Association labels "other." As you see, fire fighters have ample opportunities to see some pretty traumatic things; even slow firehouses and small volunteer departments get their share.

SECONDHAND SMOKE

Generally speaking, a *traumatic event* is a sudden, often senseless, incident that shatters the continuity of life. The cornerstone of trauma is loss. The loss can be tangible, like the loss of health or money. Or the loss can be psychological and intangible, such as the loss of a sense of safety, competence, or the ability to confidently predict what might happen next. Intangible losses seem to be the most difficult to accept. Fire fighters are not good losers. They are especially prone to blaming themselves and feeling guilty when they can't achieve what may seem impossible to the rest of us.

Trauma can be like secondhand smoke, insinuating itself into the environment, affecting everyone near and dear to the primary victim: family members, friends, coworkers, and community members. The bond that exists between fire fighters worldwide makes one fire fighter's traumatic experience the property of all. As the news spreads, fire fighters and their families everywhere wonder "What if that had been me?"

Fire fighters are compassionate people who go into the fire service primarily to help others. As much as they do help, they are frequently powerless to change the grotesque, gory, or sad situations they encounter or to comfort the inconsolable. Being close to people in pain and being unable to change their destiny—no matter how hard you try, how much you want to, or how capable you think you are—can hurt.

Having to hide your own feelings or manufacture artificial

164

emotions only adds to the difficulty. A fire captain told me that "people don't care how much we know, they care how much we care." No one—especially the victim and the victim's family—wants a fire fighter to arrive at a grisly accident and then look frightened, disgusted, incompetent, or tearful. Fire fighters must maintain an occupational persona; no matter how they feel on the inside, they need to appear friendly, competent, and compassionate on the outside. Clearly some of the stress of fire fighting comes from hiding the stress involved with the job: hiding it from the public, from fellow fire fighters, from their families, and sometimes from themselves.

One of the most difficult tasks facing fire fighters is dealing with victims' families. It's not uncommon for emergency responders to have days when they feel like they can't take any more "people pain." This is sometimes referred to as "compassion fatigue" and it affects all professional helpers. Compassion fatigue is temporary. It usually means the individual needs a break: a vacation, a different assignment, a more realistic and accepting appraisal of his or her limits, and a better balance between work and home.

FROM DISTRESS TO DISORDER: AN OVERVIEW

Stress exists along a continuum and is part of everyone's life. Positive stress actually improves performance. When you push yourself to run faster or increase the weights you lift, you make yourself stronger. That is, until you reach a point of exhaustion past which additional effort has no benefit and may be damaging.

The Pileup

Stressful events, whether negative or positive, accumulate. Your body doesn't know if you're under stress because you lost a job or because you won a promotion. The key concept is that months or years of having more demands than you can reasonably respond to results in emotional and physical wear-and-tear. Coping poorly with everyday stress is like riding around with your foot on the clutch; after a while, the clutch wears out. How long that takes depends on the condition of the clutch and how heavy your foot is.

Critical Incident Stress

Critical incident stress, also known as "acute traumatic stress," is incident-specific, that is, you can point to what caused it. It can generate considerable but temporary psychological distress lasting anywhere from a few days to many months. Sometimes it surfaces immediately, sometimes months after the event. This kind of acute stress is an occupational hazard experienced by nearly all emergency workers at some point in their careers. It is a discomfort that signals that something of great consequence outside the realm of normal experience has occurred and must be understood, coped with, and integrated into one's life. Such feelings, though uncomfortable, are neither "symptoms" of serious emotional problems nor predictors of mental illness.

WHO'S AT RISK FOR EXPERIENCING STRESS?

Recent research suggests that the best way to look at traumatic stress is to consider what factors make some people vulnerable to stress and what factors protect them. Some of these factors will be part of the incident itself and some will reside in the individual.

The Incident Itself

One of the recent assertions in trauma psychology is that there is no bona fide evidence that certain events, even horrific events like wars, are inevitably linked to enduring negative psychological outcomes. On the other hand, every fire fighter I've ever met has told me that incidents and accidents involving children or leading to the death or serious injury of another fire fighter were the most disturbing types of calls. But that doesn't mean that every such call is a predictor of serious, long-lasting symptoms or PTSD. Or that these types of calls always require immediate formal outside intervention without which there will be inescapable and serious psychological consequences.

I once attended a debriefing for several agencies that rolled on a house fire in which nine people died. Their bodies laid like logs on the front lawn under a tarpaulin until someone arrived with a makeshift tent to shield them from onlookers. Most of the dead were children who were unable to open the locked burglar-proof bars that covered the windows and the doors. The mood in the room was somber. The group was so large that there were several therapists, chaplains, and debriefers present.

As we were introducing ourselves, one of the therapists made a startling pronouncement. She said that anyone in the room who wasn't heartbroken over this incident was callous and didn't belong in the fire service. This was a preposterous overstatement. Some of those in attendance had been on the periphery of the incident or stationed at a command post around the corner. They hadn't seen or heard anything. Others were well satisfied that the incident was properly run and knew that, under the circumstances, there was little they could have done to save anyone. Some were already focused on the future, preparing to start a campaign to donate quick-release window coverings to poor families who couldn't afford them.

I would speculate that most of us were quite sad for that family and those of us with children were wondering how or if we could handle a loss of such magnitude. But we were not pathological in our range of feelings and no one in the room needed a psychologist, a chaplain, or a debriefer to dictate what feelings were normal, acceptable, or healthy.

Certain factors raise the possibility that some events, in addition to those involving children or the death or injury of a fellow fire fighter, may be more psychologically distressing than others. These factors include:

- Catastrophic loss of life
- The presence of emotionally evocative contrasting details—for example, a "Just Married" sign on the back of a car in which the newlywed occupants have been killed
- Preventable tragedies or those involving human error
- Events involving unknown causes or substances
- Conditions of prolonged uncertainty where the worst may be yet to come—for example, aftershocks in an earthquake

- Personal loss or injury
- Prolonged contact with the dead and injured
- Loss of life following extraordinary rescue efforts
- Unusual or distressing sights and sounds, such as the falling bodies at Ground Zero
- Lack of opportunity for effective action—for example, the almost totally futile search for survivors at Ground Zero
- Stressful living or working conditions—for example, poor housing, insufficient food, terrible weather, sleep deprivation

If incidents are not in and of themselves predictive of psychological well-being, what is? This is a complicated question with no easy answers. Some have suggested that it is the pileup of awful incidents that eventually gets to emergency service responders. But this does not appear to be uniformly true. The number of times emergency responders have been exposed to so-called critical incidents may actually shield them psychologically because they know that they have coped in the past and have confidence that they will cope in the future. Inexperienced fire fighters don't have that certainty, so a terrible incident may pack more of a wallop for them than it does for veteran fire fighters.

Three elements seem to raise the risk for PTSD. One is incidents that are truly terrifying—for example, fire fighters are trapped and think they are doomed. Another is incidents during which fire fighters have what is known as a "dissociative reaction," meaning that they feel as if they are in a movie or watching themselves from a distance or they can't recall much of what occurred. The third is persistent, intrusive images of the event. Fire fighters experiencing any of these three conditions, however long they have been on the job, may be at risk for psychological consequences serious enough to interfere with their ability to function at work or home. These are people for whom early intervention may be the most helpful.

The Media

Things may be more difficult if the media is involved, although fire fighters generally get good press. That's what happened to

Dave. Dave is an industrial fire fighter and volunteers in his local fire department. An explosion and fire at a grain silo in his district led to eight fatalities. The bodies were so charred that all eight fit into two body bags. By the time reporters arrived, the victims' remains had been loaded in the ambulance. It was a very grim scene, especially since many of the volunteers knew this family. When a reporter asked Dave to reload the bodies because he had missed the first "photo op," Dave was so angry at his insensitivity that he punched the reporter in the face and knocked him cold.

Knowing the Victims

Knowing the victim personally heightens the emotional impact of an incident. Imagine what it is like to respond to a fatal car wreck and find two of your children among the dead. When the victim is another fire fighter, the emotional devastation can equal that of losing a member of your biological family. The death of a coworker often leads to *survivor guilt*, an unbearable mix of elation at having survived and guilt that one's life was spared at the expense of another's death. Survivor guilt is one of the most painful human emotions.

Sometimes the victim is unknown personally, but something about him or her strikes a familiar chord. Martin, a fire fighter/paramedic, was dispatched to a scene in which a motorcyclist had flipped his bike while trying to avoid an obstacle in the road. The biker, who was neither drunk nor speeding, was dead on impact—his neck was grotesquely twisted and one side of his head had simply been "erased." Details of the incident stayed with Martin for a long time. What gave it "Velcro" was that he and the dead man had a lot in common. They were both African American, both about the same age, and both rode nearly identical motorcycles. How many times, Martin thought, have I driven this same road without my helmet, wanting to feel the wind in my hair?

Coping Styles Count

How a fire fighter copes with daily life counts a lot toward how he or she will cope with inevitable traumatic experiences. Those who are most at risk are alienated from others, insecure, dissatisfied with their jobs, and lack a sense of control over their lives. They are poor problem solvers who routinely cope with stress by denying or underestimating it. They are rugged individualists, introverts, or loners who can't ask for help and have few support systems. They may be perfectionists whose self-esteem is almost exclusively dependent upon their success at work. They may be substance abusers who use drugs, alcohol, or food to numb themselves. They often have current or past problems with depression or anxiety, or have a family history of emotional or sexual abuse.

What You Resist Persists

The important thing to remember is that bad things happen to people who may already be in some kind of trouble. Estimates are that 40–80% of people with PTSD also suffer from clinical depression. Clinically depressed people often feel too hopeless or exhausted to seek therapy. This only increases the odds that they will not recover from either condition.

Mickey is a good example of how problems in a person's private life maximize his or her risk for serious stress. Several years ago Mickey went through a series of difficult shifts, one right after the other. On his first shift, a man shot himself in the head. On his second shift, a 10-year-old boy died in a bicycle accident. On his third shift, two people were killed in a car wreck. It was as though he was surrounded by death. By his third shift, he started to feel "funny" and light-headed, like he was floating. He wanted to go home, but he couldn't leave the firehouse. All he could do was walk in circles in the parking lot and cry.

It wasn't just job-related traumatic stress that was getting to Mickey: he was going through a divorce. He and his wife had been arguing for months and he hadn't confided in anyone. When he talked about it later with a therapist, he realized that his divorce was also like a death. He had been walking around numb, feeling half-dead himself until these ghastly incidents broke through his shell and he could no longer contain his feelings. He might not have been so stressed by those three bad incidents had he not also been depressed and anxious over what was happening in his personal life.

IT'S NOT ALL IN YOUR HEAD: THE BIOCHEMISTRY OF TRAUMA

Traumatic stress is a psychobiological event that shows us how inseparable our psychological and physiological reactions are. A traumatized fire fighter may be emotionally flat at the same time his or her body is overactive. I refer to this phenomenon as "dieseling at the curb" because it reminds me of a friend's diesel engine car that choked and sputtered long after she had turned off the ignition. Traumatic events activate hundreds, maybe thousands, of neurological and biochemical changes. People who are in this "dieseling" state can be easily triggered to react as though they are still battling for their survival. They have poor tolerance for any type of physical or emotional stimulation and tend to overrespond or to withdraw in an effort to avoid overresponding. Sometimes this leads to self-medicating with drugs or alcohol, which in turn only adds to the body's already substantial burden to rid itself of stress-manufactured chemical debris.

This biochemical response is visceral and involves all our senses, particularly taste or smell. Consider the following. After two people died in a warehouse fire, Sam stopped eating barbecued hot dogs because the charred casings reminded him of the smell of burning human flesh. Darlene couldn't look at raw meat after a plane crash when she spent hours picking up body parts. Tim told me he can still taste the vomit of a baby he tried to resuscitate. Nels remembers the crunching sound he heard when he accidentally stepped through the rib cage of a body so badly burned it was indistinguishable from the surrounding debris.

POSTTRAUMATIC STRESS DISORDER

Some things are too terrible to grasp at once. Other things—naked, sputtering, indelible in their horror—are too terrible to really ever grasp at all. It is only later, in solitude, in memory, that the realization dawns: when the ashes are cold; when the mourners have departed; when

171

one looks around and finds oneself—quite to one's
surprise—in an entirely different world.
                    —DONNA TARTT, *The Secret History*

PTSD is a formally recognized mental disorder that creates major
distress and long-lasting, seriously disruptive changes in a person's life. PTSD requires medical and psychological management—the sooner the better. Some fire fighters may be more at
risk for this condition than others.

Psychologists are still arguing over the diagnosis of PTSD. It's
a complicated debate, but as I understand it some mental health
professionals think that a diagnosis of PTSD requires more than a
list of symptoms and a precipitating event. They want to include
many of the risk factors I've described in these pages. Their reasoning is that several fire fighters can experience the same event
and have similar serious symptoms, some of which, like intrusive
images, may persist for years. But only a certain percentage, probably those with risk factors, will develop full-blown PTSD. The
others can tolerate their symptoms until they fade. How large a
percentage will go on to develop PTSD or other serious emotional
problems is unknown; estimates vary from place to place, from
country to country. Some studies suggest that it is a serious widespread problem in the U.S. fire service, while others think it affects only a very small minority.

PTSD is not the end of a continuum that starts with a critical incident. It is an independent disorder. It is important to understand this and to remember that it is universal and normal
for fire fighters to show some signs of distress after a critical
event. Most will respond within weeks or months to the "tinc-
ture" of time and support from others. But fire fighters with
PTSD are "stuck": the strength of their symptoms stays the
same or intensifies. They are unresponsive to the efforts of
friends, family, and coworkers to calm them and they are sadly
unable to soothe themselves.

As it stands now, there are specific criteria for diagnosing
PTSD. A person with PTSD must have been exposed, either directly or as a witness, to an extreme trauma involving real or
threatened death or serious injury. The person's response must include intense emotions of fear, helplessness, or horror that *last*

more than one month and cause significant impairment at work, at home, or in other important areas of social function. And they must show one or more of each of the following clusters of symptoms since the trauma occurred:

Signs of reexperiencing the event

- Recurrent intrusive, distressing recollections of the event; the sufferer cannot turn memories of the incident on or off at will
- Recurrent distressing dreams of the event
- Flashbacks: acting or feeling as if the traumatic event were happening again; these can occur whether a person is sober or intoxicated
- Intense psychological distress over situations, sounds, or smells that symbolize or resemble an aspect of the traumatic event
- Intense nervous system activity (an adrenaline rush, profuse sweating, or rapid heart beat) upon exposure to things that resemble or symbolize the event, as though there existed a continuing threat to safety

Signs of numbing or avoidance behavior

- Efforts to avoid thoughts, feelings, or conversations associated with the trauma
- Efforts to avoid activities, places, or people that create memories of the trauma
- Inability to recall an important aspect of the trauma
- Markedly diminished interest or participation in significant activities
- Feeling detached or estranged from others
- An inability to express feelings
- The sense of a foreshortened future (doubt about the success of a career, marriage, children, or a normal life span)

Signs of increased arousal

- Difficulty falling or staying asleep
- Irritability or outbursts of anger
- Difficulty concentrating

- Hypervigilance
- An exaggerated startle response to loud noises or unexpected movements

PROTECTIVE FACTORS

> The best preventative is a well-managed incident conducted by a well-managed agency; this requires well-trained, well-conditioned, well-supervised, and well-grounded personnel working together to achieve a set of defined outcomes through well-prepared and well-rehearsed operations and procedures.
> —RICHARD GIST AND S. JOSEPH WOODALL,
> "Occupational Stress in the
> Contemporary Fire Service"

Caring, Competent Management

What protects fire fighters from traumatic stress is composed of many layers, just like the personal protective gear they wear to fight fires. One piece or one layer is not enough.

This much seems clear. Well-managed incidents are less stressful than poorly managed incidents regardless of the outcome. The best protection against traumatic stress is technically competent command staff who are informed, concerned, and aware of the psychological and general well-being of their subordinates, and can express their concern in an effective, helpful, and timely way.

Fire fighters and their families need resources to handle both acute and cumulative stress. Management should provide them with accessible low- or no-cost confidential mental health and substance-abuse counseling, as well as information and education regarding stress management, wellness, and maintaining personal fitness.

A Job with a Purpose

Fire fighters find solace in their work because it is guided by values and principles such as service to others, teamwork, and courage. Being engaged in a socially meaningful pursuit greater than finding personal fame or fortune promotes humility and self-esteem. It blunts the impact of negative events and helps fire fighters accept what can't be changed. Working on the front lines, where others fear to tread, allows them to distinguish between what is and what isn't important in life.

Traditions and rituals like parades, pancake breakfasts, Christmas parties, fundraising events, and toy drives define purpose in the fire service and promote a sense of belonging. When fire fighters see things they can't explain or accept, it is reassuring to locate themselves again within these familiar activities and traditions.

College philosophy professor and volunteer fire fighter Dr. Frank McClusky wrote a book about the intersection of volunteer fire fighting and philosophy. He speaks movingly of the tradition of remembering and honoring dead fire fighters from his department by placing a flag at their grave sites every Memorial Day. It gives him enormous satisfaction to be part of this ritual and to know that one day some young volunteer he has never met will do the same for him. He notes that no such dignified traditions exist to unify generations of philosophy professors.

Resilience

Psychology has changed its emphasis. Today, rather than studying what makes people sick, psychologists are looking at how people struggle well and bounce back from adversity. This field of study is called "resilience." Resilience involves more than merely surviving and it is definitely different from those faulty notions of invulnerability, rugged individualism, and self-sufficiency that have traditionally permeated the emergency services.

Resilience can be learned. It is not a trait that people have or don't have. In fact, resilience is literally built in to the fire service. It has always been there, even before psychologists gave it a name.

The features of resilience described here don't cover all the bases and are somewhat artificially separated for clarity. In real life, all these factors overlap and intertwine. Additional information about resilience can be found in the Resources.

Support Systems: The Coffee Table versus the Couch

The primary thing that keeps people resilient is caring and supportive relationships. In this regard, fire fighters who literally have two families—a work family and a real family—are twice blessed.

Fire fighters almost always prefer talking with their families and colleagues to consulting with professionals. They don't want to be seen as weak for seeking help. They don't trust that their conversations will be confidential. They are not sure how to judge whether the therapist is or isn't competent. And they question whether anyone but another fire fighter can understand what they go through and what they see.

Countless studies show that when fire fighters have front-line support from their crews and feel like they belong to a group of familiar others they show few signs of anxiety, depression, PTSD, or dissociative reactions. Social support from credible sources like other fire fighters buffers the impact of negative incidents and gives examples about how to "struggle well." Role models and heroes inspire fire fighters to see beyond the constraints of their own situations. As much as family members matter, they cannot do this in the same way, unless they are fire fighters themselves, because they can't supply the necessary technical or strategic feedback.

Smitty was a relatively new fire fighter when his crew rolled on a horse-barn fire. The structure was fully involved and fire fighters could do nothing to save 30 horses that were trapped inside. Smitty loved horses, and he was overcome with emotions as he listened to the horses dying in terror and panic. When the fire was out, the owners, many of them children who boarded their horses at this stable, arrived on scene screaming and crying in anguish. Some of them turned on the fire fighters, blaming them for not saving their beloved animals.

When he got back to the firehouse, Smitty was very quiet. He couldn't stop thinking about the scene, reviewing it over and over. His confidence was shattered and he kept second guessing himself and everyone else. Why had they not been more aggressive? How had he allowed himself to cry in public? What must his fellow fire fighters think of him now?

Questioning oneself is painful, but can be useful. Dr. Charles Figley, a trauma expert, says that in order to get past a traumatic incident a person must resolve some questions: "What happened? Why did it happen? Why did I act as I did? Why do I act as I have since? And what if it happens again?"

Patrick, who was Smitty's captain, took him aside. He talked about the decisions he made to fight the fire from outside the barn and the risks in doing otherwise. He suggested that the fire was arson, meaning it burned so fast and ferociously that the fire fighters never had a chance. Smitty had not considered arson at all. Patrick talked about his own first fatal fire and how much it affected him. He told Smitty what he learned about himself as a result—that he was a lot stronger than he had ever dreamed.

And then he gave Smitty some good advice about how best to handle folks who ragged on him for crying—which was basically to tell them to pound sand. No one, he said, goes through his or her career without shedding some tears. He told Smitty how he had cried openly standing in a field where the bodies of two boys, ages 10 and 11, were found clinging to each other after they were sucked into a drainage ditch and drowned.

Patrick didn't set out to act as an ambassador of mental health—he was just going on experience and gut instinct. But what he did for Smitty was probably more effective than what a hundred psychologists might have done. He stepped in as soon as he noticed Smitty was in trouble. First he listened, then he helped him rewrite some unreasonable beliefs and expectations he had about overcoming insurmountable odds. Finally, he normalized his reactions and helped him identify strategies to reassert control over his emotions.

This is coffee-table wisdom at it's best and one of several perks of living together—there is usually always time to sit around and debrief an incident. If someone like Smitty appears upset and not quite himself, it gets noticed. Volunteer fire fighters may have to work a little harder at this because they often go home or back to their regular jobs after a call. Even so, they may have some time to "shoot the breeze" while racking hose or restocking the medic van. Looking out for your fellow fire fighters doesn't stop when the incident is over; volunteer fire fighters are a close-knit group with strong ties to each other and to the community.

Personal Qualities: The Ability to Manage Strong Emotions and Impulses

The ability to stay calm under stress or to rapidly calm down after an emergency can be learned. It's not simply a matter of individual effort but rather the result of proper training, sufficient practice, and thorough preparation.

There is much an individual fire fighter can do to "tinker" with his or her basic wiring. "Hot reactors"—people with short fuses who go into a tailspin after minor provocation—are especially encouraged to develop self-soothing skills. It's hard to be calm emotionally until you are calm physically—both systems seem to spin out of control simultaneously. But it is your physical or neurological state that seems to be in the driver's seat.

While it's doubtful that a hard-driving Type A personality can change into a calm, unruffled, slow-moving Type B, there are many ways individual fire fighters can learn to monitor and control their physical reactions: deep-breathing techniques, yoga, progressive relaxation, or stress management, for example. Information and instruction about all these techniques are readily available in bookstores, on videotape, at community colleges, and in recreation centers.

Thoughts, Perceptions, and Reframing

One of the critical factors in how we bounce back from adversity is how we appraise or interpret an event. Human beings are meaning-making mammals: we cannot rest easy until we make sense of things. Sometimes we substitute blame for meaning: we Monday-morning quarterback each other and second-guess ourselves—I should have done this, said that, known this, been the one who died instead.

A lot of Monday-morning quarterbacking and second guessing is unfair and unreasonable. Thoughts and perceptions—especially our incorrect thoughts and distorted perceptions—trigger our emotional responses, influence our moods, affect our behavior, and determine our physical reactions. Smitty, for example, had these unwritten rules that he wasn't aware of until he talked with Patrick. His rules were: "I must always succeed" and "I must never show emotions in public." His despair over breaking these unwritten rules affected him as much as the actual incident.

Patrick guided him toward a very effective cognitive strategy that protects fire fighters from stress. He helped him reframe the situation differently. He didn't fail, the situation was not winnable from the start. *Reframing* is the ability to see something that has happened from a new and different point of view. I'm not talking about bending the truth or snowing yourself. I'm talking about accurately looking at what has occurred from a different angle in a way that you can live with.

Larry arrived at the scene of a high-impact automobile crash. There were multiple cars and multiple victims. The crews on scene were engaged in *triage*, identifying which victims needed immediate attention, which victims could wait for treatment, and which were beyond help. In one car, Larry found a young mother and her baby. The mother had no vital signs and Larry tagged her as beyond help. It was the toughest decision of his career. The baby was extricated from the crushed car and rushed to the hospital, where she died a few hours later. The baby's father made a decision to donate his daughter's organs to another child.

It was a terrible tragedy and Larry felt sad and helpless, as did all the other fire fighters on scene. With all his heart he wished things had turned out differently for this family. He wrestled with his feelings of failure and helplessness and felt angry at the random unfair way this young mother and child met their deaths. But with a little time and a lot of discussion, he was able to reframe the tragedy in a more palatable way by taking a longer, broader view of the incident. A sick infant in another state now had a new lease on life because Larry correctly assessed the situation and rushed the dying baby to the hospital before her organs were unusable. One family was destroyed, but another one was sustained.

Active Problem Solving and Communication

Fire fighters are action-oriented, take-charge problem solvers—it's what they do for a living. The ability to face problems head-on, especially emotional issues that may come up after an emergency, helps fire fighters get past the event. People who are willing to talk things over and risk expressing their feelings openly move on. Those who don't, for whatever reason, risk staying stuck.

Emmett and his crew of seasonal fire fighters were practicing water rescues in a storm when their boat capsized and they were all thrown into the freezing water. They managed to right the boat and rescue themselves. As soon as they got to shore, they headed back to base to change their clothes and get warm. Hours later Emmett got the shakes. He couldn't stop thinking about the accident and how close he had come to drowning. The thought of going back out again in the boat terrified him. "This is nuts," he said to himself, "I can't go on feeling lousy like this. I love this job."

And then he had a brainstorm. He gathered the team around the coffee table and started a conversation about the day's events. When he worked up enough nerve he made a serious disclosure. "I don't know about you guys," he said, "but I thought I was going to die out there today and I doubt I'm the only one who felt that way." And he wasn't. One by one each crew member talked about how frightened he had been, scared of never seeing his family again, angry at dying so young, sad to feel his life was incomplete. It was an amazing conversation. It brought the team together for having shared both the experience and the discussion afterward. Next day, everyone was prepared to go out on the boat and do it all over again.

One of the great benefits of talking things over with trusted friends and family is that in times of uncertainty you get to compare your situation with that of others. You get to assess what's "normal" or acceptable and how you stand relative to the rest. Until Emmett and his crew talked, each one felt isolated, as though he was the only one with such feelings. Once everyone compared notes, it became obvious that this was a common experience, that no one needed to be ashamed about it, and that there was nothing wrong about thinking that way.

Distancing

Fire fighters need to be able to distance themselves from victims, which sounds harsh, but really isn't. Without that firewall—a zen-like emotional detachment—fire fighters risk being so over-come with emotion that they can't function effectively during or after a traumatic incident. The ability to focus and stay on-task was what helped fire fighters at Ground Zero to keep searching despite their broken hearts.

As I said earlier, fire fighters distance themselves from trauma in many ways, some of which their families and the public may find hard to understand, such as humor or an obsessive interest in the gruesome details. Some are consoled by religion. They dis-tance themselves from the trauma by putting things in God's hands, not their own. Others are tough-minded and conclude that life has it's own plan: when your number's up, your number's up. They don't spend a lot of time thinking about victims as people, because that would close the distance.

Keeping distance is a particular challenge for volunteers who work in small communities where everyone knows everyone else. In one day, a volunteer fire fighter might run into the widow of a heart attack victim or the family of a boy saved from drowning. The widow might cry when she sees the fire fighter and the boy's family might be all smiles and gratitude.

Playing a Poor Hand Well: Finding the Challenge in Adversity

Every life, at some points, must be tested by adversity. We must face losses we can neither prevent nor reverse, confront threats we can never fully neutralize, and master challenges both sought and assumed. With adversity come sorrow and distress, but from its mastery come strength, character, and resolve.

—RICHARD GIST

Resilient people are optimistic. They are also realistic and practi-cal. They accept emotions and trauma as the cost of doing busi-ness and deal with them. They value what they have—friends, family, jobs, religious beliefs, faith in humanity—over what they might want but never get: money, fame, a more perfect world. They are confident in their abilities, and have a positive view of themselves. When things are tough, they can count on themselves to get past the rough spots. They accept their limits gracefully, of-ten with humor, even while they wish they didn't have them. Doesn't that sound like a lot of fire fighters you know?

POSTTRAUMATIC GROWTH

> Life breaks everyone, and afterwards many are strong at
> the broken places.
> —ERNEST HEMINGWAY, *A Farewell to Arms*

When I talk to new fire fighters I deliver a sermonette. I tell them, "This job will change you, but it doesn't have to damage you." I go on to explain that not all negative experiences have negative consequences. I warn them that they will see some dreadful stuff in their careers and learn things about people they wish they didn't know. But I also assure them that *if* they take as good care of themselves as they do of their equipment and *if* they receive the support they deserve, most of the awful things they see will actually increase their compassion for the human condition, fortify their self-esteem for doing tough and important work, and reinforce the pride they have in their professional family.

Enduring and surviving harrowing life experiences is a source of pride for fire fighters. Few people can do what they do. What most of us consider a crisis, they consider a challenge. I remember walking up Third Avenue in New York City with my brother, Richard, a volunteer fire fighter from California. Smoke was billowing out of the second story of a four-story brownstone. Quick as a wink, my brother ran around the corner to the front door of the building and began hitting all the intercom buzzers to tell people their building was on fire. When someone popped the door open, he ran inside and upstairs knocking on doors and shouting for people to leave. I stood on the street holding the front door open for the tenants as they raced out.

It seemed like an eternity before my brother reappeared out of the smoke. By this time the fire department had arrived and we walked away without any thanks or recognition. My brother didn't need any. Feeling good about his actions was recognition enough. While this incident wasn't by any means traumatic, it proves a point made by authors Vickie Taylor and Sybil Wolin who said that "when things are at their worst, firefighters are at their best."

In the ancient art of Chinese calligraphy the word "crisis" is represented as a blending of danger and opportunity. This is precisely what modern science is now claiming. Every traumatic incident can be an opportunity for growth. If you only ask trauma victims about their negative reactions or judge everyone by the folks who seek psychological assistance, you get a picture that is skewed toward the morose. When you reframe the picture and ask trauma survivors what they gained from their experiences, a different picture emerges.

According to trauma researchers Lawrence Calhoun and Richard Tedeschi, trauma survivors report the following:

Changes in themselves

- Increased self-confidence in coping with the future—after what they have been through, they feel capable of facing just about anything
- Increased self-reliance
- A sense of being vulnerable—now they know for sure that bad things happen—yet they feel stronger for having survived

Changes in their relationships with others

- Public personas are dropped; relationships with others are deepened and made more intimate by talking and self-disclosure
- An increased sense of compassion for the suffering of others and connection to humanity in general

Changes in their spirituality and orientation to life

- A new set of life priorities
- An increased appreciation for life and for the people in one's life.
- More emphasis on the importance of spirituality, philosophy, or religion in their lives

Not every trauma victim reports positive posttraumatic changes, but so many do that a distinct pattern has formed. Universal themes of posttraumatic growth are seen in all kinds of survivors, including first responders like fire fighters. This doesn't mean that fire fighters won't suffer or struggle when they experience something traumatic, but it does strongly suggest that there is much to be salvaged from a bad situation. Surviving a traumatic incident can make you stronger for having incorporated a powerful event into your life. It can connect you more deeply with others and more deeply with parts of yourself you may not have known existed. (Tips for dealing with trauma are at the end of Chapter 11.)

CHAPTER 11

Treating Traumatic Stress
Help for Individuals and Families

> Exposure to critical incidents is not only unavoidable in fire
> and rescue work; it is the essence of the enterprise.
> —RICHARD GIST and S. JOSEPH WOODALL,
> "There Are No Simple Solutions to Complex Problems"

The controversy in trauma psychology really heats up around the issue of intervention and treatment. At the center of the controversy is the efficacy of critical incident stress debriefings. *Debriefings* are structured group or individual conversations, often compulsory, that are scheduled for emergency responders shortly following a critical incident. They are designed to elicit facts and emotions, process their impact, share information, normalize responses, and educate the participants about traumatic stress.

The intention of critical incident debriefings is honorable: to reduce suffering and prevent serious psychological consequences like PTSD. What is coming into question, however, is the science behind this technology and the claims made for its effectiveness.

Behavioral scientists around the world have a range of opinions about the widespread use of debriefings. Some studies suggest that debriefings may actually damage at-risk participants, leaving them worse off than if they had received no intervention at all. Others assert that debriefings are overly negative: they pathologize critical incidents, manufacture dire prophecies, and reinforce notions of illness. Critics of debriefings contend that it is more accurate to propose that people are resilient—most of us will bounce back from adversity using our own resources rather than depending on professionals or outsiders.

Other commentators maintain that debriefings have no effect at all on relieving or preventing postincident psychological consequences. They argue that debriefings are a waste of time and money for everyone but the employers who are trying to protect themselves against stress disability claims and the people who profit either from conducting debriefings or from training debriefers.

The effectiveness of debriefings is difficult to study because there is a lack of uniformity in how and when they are conducted, who facilitates them, who attends, and under what conditions. To complicate matters further, people who conduct or participate in debriefings often have quite positive feelings about their experiences. This is puzzling in light of the negative findings. Dr. Richard Gist, special assistant to the fire chief in Kansas City, Missouri, and an outspoken critic of the debriefing "industry," describes this paradox as follows:

> People appreciate warm doughnuts, [they] like the folks who hand 'em out, and generally say that they really hit the spot . . . but that doesn't make them even remotely nutritious. . . . We're not saying that folks shouldn't try to help or that all approaches to help are likely to prove harmful—but we are saying that help shouldn't be shoved down throats, and that there's no evidence to support the contention that everyone has to emote or that repression will invariably lead to problems.

Until the debate is settled the International Society for Traumatic Stress Studies (ISTSS) recommends that participation in debriefings should be voluntary; that all providers should be experienced, well-trained practitioners; that debriefings should focus on screening, education, and support rather than on revisiting the details of the incident; that potential participants should be evaluated by a trained practitioner prior to debriefing, and that further research be conducted to compare debriefings with alternative early interventions. Other groups have recommended discontinuing debriefings entirely.

WHAT WORKS

Cognitive-Behavioral Therapy

This promising, well-documented therapeutic approach involves a short series of individual appointments, each lasting from 60 to 90 minutes. During the treatment victims are educated about traumatic reactions, taught progressive muscle relaxation, exposed in a systematic manner to visual memories of the traumatic incident, helped to restructure beliefs they may hold about themselves or the incident, and gradually reintroduced to situations they may be avoiding. Clients are active participants—expect to do homework.

Medication

Stress hormones help a person cope in a critical situation, but they may also make the memory of that situation more intense and/or induce flashbacks, especially if that person has a genetic predisposition toward a chemical imbalance in the production of these hormones. For this reason, it is critically important to interrupt the body's continued outpouring of stress-related hormones such as adrenaline as soon after the incident as possible. Fire fighters who are "dieseling" hard—their resting heart rates may be above 90 beats per minute—or who have experienced dissociative reactions may find relief with certain types of medication such as b-blocker propanolol or antidepressants. Medication helps enormously in both acute and chronic reactions. Your family doctor can prescribe medication, or better still, refer you to a specialist.

Exercise

Exercise is a tried-and-true antidote for stress, even serious stress. Some researchers think it is as effective as antidepressants in fighting depression. Movement flushes those stress chemicals through your body. But keep your exercise goals realistic and manageable: you're more apt to consistently walk your dog three times a week than you are to get up everyday at 5:00 A.M. to train for a marathon. Some exercise calms and soothes. Yoga, for example, includes deep breathing and meditation, benefitting the student physically and emotionally.

Eye Movement and Desensitization Reprocessing (EMDR)

This intervention is still considered experimental by many. It involves visualizing the critical incident while rapidly moving one's eyes in accordance with instructions from a trained practitioner. Proponents claim that it produces rapid results within a few sessions. Detractors debunk their claims as self-serving bad science. Those in the middle speculate that the eye movement is basically irrelevant and that the active ingredient comes with helping the client focus on aspects of the experience he or she may have been avoiding.

Psychotherapy

People at risk for PTSD often concurrently struggle with other psychological conditions such as anxiety or depression. If your postincident symptoms don't abate within 30 days or less, consider seeking psychological help from a mental health professional who specializes in the treatment of traumatic stress *and* is familiar with the fire service culture.

Is it always necessary to work with a public safety psychologist? That would depend on the problem. Most everyone has aging parents, adolescent children, financial problems, marital woes, trouble quitting smoking, and so on at some point in their life. But if your problems are directly related to your work, then you may feel most comfortable consulting with someone who understands and has experience working with emergency responders (see Chapter 14). Psychotherapists can also help you manage your emotions by teaching you self-hypnosis, meditation, progressive relaxation, and so on.

Expressing Yourself

Trauma can scare us speechless. On the other hand, staying healthy seems to require translating our experiences into language. Writing or "journaling" have been shown to positively influence immune system functioning, improve our moods, and reduce stress. Writing in a private diary allows you to express yourself at your own pace without any pressure to say or think the "right" thing. Writing helps you organize your thoughts as well as your memories of an event. It can be especially helpful in the weeks following a trauma when you or the people around you may be "burned out" on talking or listening. If you've gone through a traumatic experience or a difficult time, try writing your thoughts in a journal once a week for a month.

Creating a Mission

Being part of something larger than oneself is a hallmark of a resilient person. One of the ways people recover from trauma is to find a way to keep others from similar suffering. Candy Lightener, the founder of Mothers Against Drunk Driving, used her own tragic loss to start a national organization that has strongly influenced public policy. The events of 9/11 produced countless examples of how survivors' missions, large or small, helped heal individuals, families, and communities.

Distraction

Escaping your problems has gotten a bad rap; I know people who feel guilty if they aren't ruminating over their tragedies. Actually, rumination and an obsessive interest in the negative aspects of life are signs of serious emotional problems. This is different from getting good information about what happened. The fire service is generally very good at investigating critical incidents and publicizing the details.

So, go ahead, distract yourself: turn off the TV, especially the TV news, watch a funny movie, take your family on a hike, make soup, read a really good book, pull weeds, or play games with your kids. Give yourself a little temporary relief with something new and engaging to occupy your thoughts. This is not the same as numbing yourself with alcohol or losing yourself in an affair.

Sometimes distraction assumes the form of taking time off from work or changing jobs within the department. There is no shame in requesting either if you need it, especially when your request is made in the service of sustaining your career.

FAMILIES AND TRAUMA

The mutual love and compassion of family is often the single-most significant factor in successfully coping with traumatic stress. Families are "holding environments," safe places where you can let down your defenses. Family members are the people you can turn to when you need practical assistance or someone to pinch-hit for you while you recover from a traumatic experience. Families are true "first responders"—the first to spot sleeping problems, changes in appetite or mood, excessive use of alcohol, and so on. Families offer emotional as well as practical support. As a family, you have a shared history, meaning that you have experienced each other in multiple roles and can reference a list of behaviors, accomplishments, and positive qualities that can fortify your loved one's self-esteem, especially if he or she is feeling guilty or responsible. This goes a long way toward reassuring sufferers that one sin is *not* worth a thousand good deeds and that their behavior at work is separate from who they are as people.

Mark had had an absolutely terrible day. He responded to a multiple-fatality fire in which several children were badly burned, including an infant. He tried to perform CPR on the infant, and, as he did, the baby's face came off in his hands. His captain let the whole team leave early. When Mark came home, his wife, Bonnie, could easily see that he was upset. He managed to tell her the story. While it was hard to listen to, she did just that. She was unable to change what happened, of course, but she could reassure Mark that he did his best under horrible circumstances.

Mark was apologetic about burdening her with the details, especially because he had his entire crew and his captain to talk to. But still, Bonnie was his intimate, the person with whom he shared everything. Having her "witness" this most excruciating call was especially helpful. So was the back rub she offered. Making supper and cleaning up together afterward brought some normalcy back into Mark's life. He appreciated Bonnie's quiet presence and her understanding that he didn't feel much like talking for the rest of the evening.

COMPASSION: YOUR ACHILLES HEEL

> Whatever level of emotional pain a firefighter may be willing to endure in the course of his/her duties, there appears little justification for expecting a spouse, relative or friend to fall victim to the pressures of "offloading" that may follow a difficult incident. . . . Spouses and friends may be providing an essential service to the country's firefighters with no payment, training or support. Potentially they face the kind of emotional pressures for which mental health professionals are provided with specialized training and support.
> —JOHN DURKIN AND DEBRA A. BEKERIAN,
> *Psychological Resilience to Stress in Firefighters*

Living with someone who has been through a traumatic experience is hard. It costs you something to provide your loved one with the support he or she needs. That's why it's important to protect yourself from damage while reaching out to someone else. The best protection is to understand trauma and have a good sense of what you can and cannot realistically do to help. It's also crucial to be prepared and have your own support systems. During traumatic times, the fire fighter you love may be so caught up in the exceptional incident that he or she has little to give back by way of thanks or by way of participating in ordinary family life.

Bonnie was prepared. It was hard for her to watch Mark suffering and she felt badly that she couldn't do more to comfort him. But she had learned over the years to be patient—not to push him or to expect too much from herself. She knew that in time things would even out and get better. She actually learned to enjoy those times when Mark shared awful things from work because he was more loving, emotional, and communicative than usual. This was not always true for some of her friends who complained that their spouses were withdrawn, irritable, and self-centered after a bad incident.

That's what happened to Martha, whose husband, Tom, went to Ground Zero to help in the recovery effort. He returned home discouraged and deeply depressed by his failure to find even one intact body. The community where they lived considered Tom and his coworkers to be heroes. They sponsored parades and held barbecues in their honor. Tom wasn't sleeping or eating well. He was moody and wouldn't talk to Martha even though she begged him to talk to her. He and Martha attended a few crisis intervention groups, but they didn't help. The only thing that seemed to give him relief was talking to community groups and telling his story over and over—the same story he couldn't bear to tell at home.

Martha went to all of Tom's presentations. It was the only way she could learn about his experiences at Ground Zero. She felt like a failure as a wife because she couldn't force Tom to confide in her and she was terrified that he would crack up on the first anniversary of the disaster. She was suffering almost as much as him, and her emotional well-being was equally in jeopardy.

CHILDREN AND TRAUMA

Children are the most vulnerable family members because they are still learning how to manage their emotions. Even adolescents, no matter how mature they appear to be, need help managing the social or psychological consequences of traumatic stress.

Children respond to family stress according to age. Young children are concerned with issues of separation and safety and they need assistance putting their feelings into words. As we now know, translating trauma into language is how we resolve or soften the experience. Older children, especially teens, are sensitive to being in the spotlight and being different from their friends.

Job-related trauma comes home to children in several ways. Fire fighters can be overly concerned and restrictive with their children because they have seen too many tragic events involving kids. Others may be less than sympathetic because their children's problems pale in comparison to what fire fighters encounter at work.

How children react when job-related trauma comes home frequently depends on how you as parents are reacting. Indeed, children tend to imitate adults and will react more to their parents' emotional reactions than to the event itself.

Children of parents who hold public safety jobs have a unique challenge. They have to deal with the certain knowledge that in the event of a disaster, natural or man-made, their parent or parents will most likely be at work or called back to the job. This awareness has been made profoundly real by the events of 9/11.

Ellyn and Lou thought they had all their bases covered after 9/11. Lou is a battalion chief and Ellyn is a police officer. They were both at home with their children, Julie, age 14, and Sonny, age 9, on September 11th. Ellyn was on medical leave and Lou was on his four days off. Like many families, they were glued to the TV.

Julie and Sonny seemed to settle back into their usual routines until Ellyn returned to work after New Year's. On her first shift back she got a frantic phone call from Julie. Sonny had had a "complete meltdown" at school. He was in the nurse's office totally hysterical, crying that he wanted to kill himself because "it's going to happen again and my parents are going to die."

Lou and Ellyn raced to school and brought Sonny home, where he continued to sob for hours and plead with Ellyn to quit work. He didn't want to return to class and begged his parents to school him at home. They called a family counselor. After much deliberation, Ellyn took an extended unpaid leave of absence and ultimately resigned her job. She loved her work, but Sonny needed her more.

Sonny's better now, although still fragile and still in counseling. In retrospect, both Lou and Ellyn wished they had talked more and watched less TV. Lou regrets being so tied up in work that he missed some signs that Sonny was in trouble. Neither he nor Ellyn paid attention to his school performance. They were astonished to learn later that his grades had dropped significantly after 9/11 and that other children were taunting him, telling him that his parents would be killed in another terrorist attack.

While they wish Sonny had been spared such suffering, there have been some positive outcomes to this crisis. Therapy has brought the family closer; they are more openly affectionate and appreciative of each other. They are also more honest. Sonny is free to be himself and not act tougher or more grown-up than he feels. Julie no longer has to shoulder as much responsibility for her younger brother. It's been an effort. They've had to shuffle priorities and trim the budget in order to strengthen their family bonds. But that's what it takes to guide children through times of uncertainty.

Signs of Trouble

The following behaviors are typical of the ways children respond to trauma. If they persist unabated for several weeks, consider getting professional consultation.

Temper Tantrums

Anger, hostility, tantrums, mood swings, and other unruly behavior may be a sign that your child is feeling afraid or helpless. Try to uncover what is going on rather than react. Help your child find other ways to express feelings. Encourage young children to relieve tension using hand puppets, finger paints, soft toys, or pillows they can hit. Older children can talk things out, write stories or poems, or create a journal. They can write letters they never intend to mail or make up newspaper stories starring themselves and their families.

Aches and Pains

When children can't put words to their feelings, they may turn these feelings into a variety of physical ailments for which there is no medical cause. Sometimes this is a ruse to stay home from school because they can't bear being apart from Mom or Dad. Get them to talk, acknowledge that things are rough, then gently insist they continue their normal routines and responsibilities.

Guilt and Responsibility

Kids have an uncanny way of assuming responsibility for things over which they have no control. Children of divorce need repeated reassurances that the divorce is not their fault. So it goes with children of public safety professionals who may worry that Mom or Dad was hurt because they forgot to say their prayers or kiss them good-bye.

Remind your children that thoughts are not the same as facts. Just because you feel guilty doesn't mean you did something wrong; just because you're afraid doesn't mean there is truly something to fear.

Bedtime Troubles

Children who are upset or anxious often have trouble sleeping or going to bed on time. Deal with bedtime troubles as soon as possible because restoring normal routines is comforting. Bedtime troubles can be hard to fix. Moreover, they are a misery for parents who need quiet time for themselves. The following guidelines may help.

- It's okay to postpone bedtime when a child is anxious and wants to talk. But limit the delays. Use a timer.
- If your children are afraid to sleep alone, spend some extra time in their bedrooms. If that doesn't help, you can allow your children to sleep on a mattress on the floor of your bedroom or with a sibling. But this arrangement shouldn't last longer than three or four days and you should establish this limit in advance.
- Make certain you're not inadvertently communicating fears of your own. Ask yourself, do I need my child's company in the bedroom as much as he or she needs mine?
- Get your child a night light or leave the closet light on. Leave the door ajar. Buy him or her a big stuffed animal to sleep with.
- Make sure you're spending enough time with your child during the day. Children need *quantity* time in order to have *quality* time.
- If your child comes out of her room, calmly walk her back to bed and reassure her that you're close by. You need to set limits, but getting angry, punishing, spanking, or shouting rarely helps.
- If your children have nightmares, encourage them to draw their nightmares in a storybook. Help them fight back. Teach them to stand up to their night-time monsters and order them out of their dreams.

School Phobias and Problems

Some children, like Sonny, are so afraid of being separated from their parents that they refuse to go to school. School phobias can be hard to reverse, so it is important to stand firm on this. Try to get to the bottom of what's bothering your child—for example, is he afraid to let Mom or Dad out of his sight or is he being teased or talked about? If the problem is with his classmates—kids can be terribly insensitive—try coaching him about what to say to his friends. Rehearse and role-play responses that increase your child's social confidence.

Talk to your children's teachers. They need to know that your kids are under stress and may be distracted or have trouble concentrating. Advise teachers how to be helpful and what to tell other students, if anything. Alert school counselors and find a safe haven in school—a responsible, empathic adult who can provide a quiet space for your child.

If your children are having trouble concentrating or completing homework, make some reasonable, short-term allowances. Provide help, if needed. Break study time into smaller segments; your children may be able to concentrate for 15 but not for 30 minutes. Use breaks and time-out periods to defuse tension and anxiety. Give your children a timer and let them set it themselves. Stress affects our ability to think clearly; keep your expectations reasonable and accept "good enough" schoolwork for the time being.

Fears and Avoidant Behavior

Frightened children may want to avoid the things that scare them; sometimes even the mention of something fearful is upsetting. Time and a lot of authentic reassurance helps. In severe cases your child may need professional help.

Never give false reassurances you can't guarantee such as "nothing bad will ever happen to your father or me." Instead, talk to children, in child terms, about what will occur in a disaster: who will take care of them, where they will sleep, what toys they can bring, and so on.

Prepare a disaster plan. Include plans for communicating

with each other. Afterward, everyone will need to talk about how he or she felt and what happened to them during the separation or the crisis. Small children can draw pictures or act out their experiences with hand puppets or toys. Or they can dictate their stories while you write them down in a blank book to which you can later add pictures. Be sure to include positive memories—how brave or how helpful your child was, what he learned and so on— along with the scary ones.

Monitor and/or restrict your children's TV viewing. Children, like adults, need accurate information given in palatable doses in child-appropriate language. And they need an adult to help them understand what they see and hear. The barrage of instant replays of airplanes crashing into the World Trade Center, the Pentagon, and the field in Pennsylvania left some children with the impression that hundreds of planes were crashing all over the United States.

Regressive Behavior

It is universal for traumatized children to revert to behaviors they have outgrown. Potty-trained kids may start wetting their beds again. They may be needy, clingy, and demand to be fed or held. They may whine, cry, and suck their thumbs. Older children who have learned to do for themselves may need Mom's or Dad's help again.

These are temporary stress reactions that will soon pass. While childish behavior is hard to take, avoid ridiculing it. Make an effort, instead, to reward and acknowledge mature behavior when it occurs. Children respond to praise and positive guidance.

WHEN TO GET PROFESSIONAL HELP

If the changes you observe in your children don't pass or diminish in intensity or frequency in about four weeks, consider consulting your pediatrician. This is especially important if your child has become excessively hypervigilant or fearful or engages in negative repetitive play about the incident.

Serious acting out is reason to seek consultation, as are any radical changes in your children's moods, behaviors, or basic patterns of sleeping and eating. Consultation is also in order if your children are emotionally constricted, listless, socially withdrawn, or disinterested in their usual activities. Aggressive acting out, a major loss of appetite accompanied by weight loss, and suicidal or homicidal thoughts or threats require *immediate* professional attention.

Tips for Coping with Traumatic Stress

- Establish reasonable goals for what posttrauma life will look like. Make them specific, measurable, and achievable. Wanting to entertain friends once a month is a realistic and measurable goal. Wanting everything to be the way it was and for all of you to be happy again is an understandable but not a realistic goal. Allow time for your family and yourself to integrate what has happened and adjust to the "new normal."
- Fire fighters: Don't go it alone. Seek professional help if you:
  - Are experiencing severe mood swings
  - Can't sleep for days on end
  - Have repeated nightmares
  - Have angry or violent outbursts
  - Are depressed, guilt-ridden, or suicidal
  - Start using alcohol or other drugs to excess
  - Are not back to normal after four weeks

- Pay attention to your dreams and to the "movies" and dialogues that go on in your head. They are clues to what you are feeling.
- Learn all you can about posttraumatic stress and secondary trauma. Accept that strong emotions are the cost of doing business and not a sure sign of emotional breakdown.
- Focus on what went right. Acknowledge good coping and struggling well.
- Family or spouses: If *you* need professional help, get it. Your fire fighter may have employee assistance benefits that include free confidential visits for family members. Or your

(*continued from previous page*)

medical insurance may provide for mental health counseling (see Chapter 14).

- Don't bottle up your feelings. Keep a journal, write letters you never mail, go online and pour your heart out to other fire fighters and fire fighter spouses (see Resources).

- Monitor the way you talk to yourself. Your interpretation of a problem determines your response. For instance, if your mate is unaffectionate and disinterested in sex, don't assume it is because you are unlovable or unattractive. His or her disinterest may have little to do with you and everything to do with traumatic stress. Challenge your negative assumptions. Talk to your spouse.

- Consult your department chaplain or peer support personnel. If your department doesn't have programs like these available to families, use your own experience to start one.

CHAPTER 12

Fire Fighters in Hot Water

Alcoholism, Arson, Divorce, and Infidelity

It's May 16, 2003. The headlines on Firehouse.com are a hodge-podge of good and bad news: "Fire fighters Jailed for Multiple Arsons"; "Cocaine Bust Snags NY [Fire] Chief"; "Police Probe Ohio [Fire] Captain for Links to Other Assaults"; "Tennessee Fire fighter Donates Kidney to Fellow Fire fighter"; and "Twenty-Five Rescued from English Pub Arson."

Ordinarily it's the acts of service and sacrifice that make "front-page" news in the fire service press. When bad news makes headlines, it's jarring. "How could this happen?", fire fighter families wonder. "How often?" and "What if it happened to us?"

As I did research for this book, I encountered a number of pernicious stereotypes about fire fighters, not just from the public but, remarkably, from fire fighters themselves. These stereotypes ranged along a continuum. At one end I heard that fire fighters are superhuman heroes. At the other end, I was told that they are philandering "boozers" bound for divorce. Some months into my work several high-profile incidents and a TV drama based on a popular book added another negative to the list: the fire fighter arsonist.

Stereotypes are simplistic ways to pigeon-hole and label large groups of people as though they were all the same. At the very least they are insulting. At the worst they distort and damage the truth, unnecessarily raising anxiety and reducing our ability to confidently predict the future.

It's just as harmful to overinflate a problem as it is to ignore its existence. I grouped the subjects in this chapter together to give families an even-handed look at the probability that such extreme behaviors will affect them personally. And if they do, I've provided some suggestions about how best to react.

ALCOHOLISM AND SUBSTANCE ABUSE

> Fire fighters never die, they just eat smoke and drink fire water.
>
> —ANONYMOUS

No one really knows how widespread alcoholism and alcohol abuse are in the fire service. Even less is known about drug use. Fire fighters rarely come forward and admit to such troubles, suggesting that the problem may be more extensive than generally acknowledged. Sadly, it takes alcohol-related tragedies—like the deaths of eight paid on-call fire fighters or the death of a 16-year-old volunteer—to bring the issue to the surface.

The Basic Facts

More than half of all adult Americans drink alcohol. Nearly 10% will experience some problems with alcoholism and most of those will be men. Alcohol problems are highest among young people ages 18–29. Children who start drinking at age 14 or younger greatly increase the chances that they will have alcohol problems later in life. Problem drinking is also associated with emotional conditions such as depression, anxiety, and PTSD.

Individuals with a family history of alcoholism face significant risk. They are not doomed to be alcoholics—in fact more than half are not—but they are four times more likely than the general population to be problem drinkers or to have other emotional or behavioral problems. Genes are not the only contributing factor. Growing up in a family with an alcoholic parent or parents can be psychologically damaging, especially when accompanied by violence, divorce, or financial or emotional instability.

Alcoholics can hold challenging jobs and function well for years before their work performance is noticeably affected. There is great variety in alcohol abuse. Some people get drunk every day, others only on the weekends, and some stay sober for months and then go on a binge. The one thing we know for sure is that alcoholism is a disease for which recovery is guaranteed *if* the alcoholic starts and then stays with a recovery program.

Risk Factors at Work

Research on prevalence rates of alcoholism among urban fire fighters range from a low of 18–30% and a high of 42% following exposure to death and injury. One study of 181 fire fighters who responded to the Oklahoma City bombing found low rates of PTSD (13%) and high rates of alcohol abuse/dependence (47%.) The second-most reported postbombing coping strategy—after seeking interpersonal support—was drinking alcohol.

When you consider the fire service as a whole, it's easy to see how the risk factors pile up. It's a male-dominated workforce that's routinely exposed to significant levels of on-the-job stress and trauma. There is chronic tension waiting for something to happen or filling the hours spent waiting. Sleep problems are common and fire fighters may mistakenly use alcohol as a sleep aid ("mistakenly" because alcohol actually interferes with sleep). Off-duty socializing and drinking are common, as they are in most occupations requiring on-the-job teamwork. Shift work or long hours spent on the job further increase dependence on co-workers and can isolate fire fighters from their families and their non-fire-fighting companions. Finally, some fire fighters may be perilously overinvested in their work, meaning that their self-esteem is dependent on the job. This makes them more vulnerable to peer pressure.

In some places alcohol is bound up with the social mission fire departments have in their communities. Many volunteer departments, for example, serve as clubhouses for their members and derive a substantial percentage of their funding from renting out the firehouse for social events from weddings to wakes.

But the biggest risk factor of all is that drinking to socialize, relax, or celebrate is deeply entrenched in fire service tradition. A cold beer after a hot fire is a reward for working hard, a way to "let your hair down," and to build bonds with your crew. This tradition is slowly changing, but not without a fight.

Many departments, career and volunteer, have implemented zero tolerance for drinking on the job and some have begun random testing for drugs and alcohol. A lot of fire fighters consider firehouses their second homes, not their workplaces, and feel entitled to the same comforts they have in their own houses. (Some make the same argument about having pornography on the premises.) It's ironic that people who frequently see the tragic results of alcohol-related accidents would be willing to drink on the job or let others do the same. And it's absurd to think that fire fighters can encourage each other to drink, but not become drunks.

The consequences of alcoholism extend far beyond the anguish and misery endured by individuals and their families. In a profession based on teamwork and public trust, every alcohol-related accident, crime, or instance of negligent or outrageous behavior disgraces the fire service and tarnishes fire fighters' normally sterling reputations.

Barney's Story

Barney, age 24, was married with two children when he joined the fire service. He had worked in construction since high school. His wife, Belle, was a bank manager. Belle accepted Barney's new life, and even welcomed the security of a regular job not dependent on the weather. But it didn't take long before the nightlife and the long hours hanging with the fellows got to her. She especially hated the banquets where her husband and his coworkers got "shit-faced" on free booze, including the battalion chief.

Things got worse when Barney became active in his union. They fought a lot; he took the labor side and she argued for management. But what upset her most was the beer drinking at union meetings, after which Barney and the other fire fighters would adjourn to a local club and drink until closing time. She worried because he was driving home drunk and she was angry because he needed the entire next day to sober up.

It didn't take long before Barney's work performance suffered. He needed a beer and a joint before bed and then again first thing in the morning just to feel normal. At times he came to work so hungover that he would nap in his rig (engine) just so he wouldn't be left behind when a call came in. Everybody knew about it, but drinking was so common in his firehouse—for years the refrigerator had been stocked with beer—and Barney was so popular no one dared "turn him in."

Covering for Barney was well intended. It's what the "brotherhood" does for each other as a gesture of solidarity. No one consciously tried to collude with him, but in their attempts to protect Barney they rationalized his behavior and reinforced his denial. "He's a good guy with a problem," they said. "Too bad his bitchy wife is driving him to drink." Covering was also self-serving. If someone "ratted" on Barney, couldn't he rat on them?

When a nurse at the local ER told the company officer that she thought Barney had been drinking at work, he told her that "it was not his job to smell people's breath." He too was aware of the problem but he had neither the training nor the courage to confront the situation.

By now it was Barney's habit to drink on the way to work to medicate his anxiety. His hands were beginning to shake and he was having secret panic attacks at work. Things were no better at home: Belle and the children had moved out. Four blocks from the firehouse Barney got into a minor car accident. The first officer on the scene knew Barney and wrote him a ticket rather than arrest him for driving under the influence.

It didn't take much for the driver of the other car to figure out that Barney was a fire fighter—he had department decals all over his truck and was wearing a department sweatshirt—nor long for her to complain to the fire chief. Barney was sure his career was over; he'd lost his family and now he was going to lose his job. To his surprise, the chief offered him a deal: he could keep his job if he would check into a 28-day residential program, agree to random drug and alcohol screening, and promise to attend department-sponsored Alcoholics Anonymous (AA) meetings run by fire fighters who were themselves recovering alcoholics.

When Barney returned to work a month later he had another surprise. His crew had strung urine cups all over the station like

Christmas-tree lights. When he was drinking, he would have thought that this was funny, but now that he was fighting to maintain sobriety the joke fell flat.

Recovery was harder than he had anticipated. He found it difficult to shake his reputation as a drinker and felt pressure to change back to being the "old Barney." His buddies repeatedly invited him to "party." They handed him beers. If he took a nap at work, he was teased about being hungover. Now that he was clean and sober, he suspected that his drinking buddies didn't trust him anymore. The only fire fighters he felt comfortable with were members of his recovery group. Eventually he transferred stations. He and Belle started counseling and reconciled after Barney had three years of sobriety. Belle understood that Barney alone was responsible for controlling his drinking, but she never stopped resenting the fire department for encouraging him to drink.

WHO IS AN ALCOHOLIC?

Use the following checklist published by the National Institute on Alcohol Abuse and Alcoholism (see Resources) to determine whether you or someone close to you has a drinking problem:

1. Have you ever felt you should cut down on your drinking? Y/N
2. Have people annoyed you by criticizing your drinking? Y/N
3. Have you ever felt bad or guilty about your drinking? Y/N
4. Have you ever had a drink first thing in the morning to steady your nerves or to get rid of a hangover? Y/N

One "Yes" suggests a possible problem. More than one "Yes" means a probable problem and sends a strong signal: you or your loved one should consult your doctor or other health care provider right away to discuss the issue and make a plan of action. There are many strategies for dealing with problem drinking including a combination of counseling, medication, and self-help groups.

Do You Love an Alcoholic?

It's hard to know what to do when someone you love and care about is addicted to alcohol or drugs. When are you being helpful and when are you helping the drinker to cover his mistakes or to minimize her responsibility? There are no pat answers; every family is challenged differently.

Living with an alcoholic is stressful. I included this 20-question quiz from Al-Anon in my first book. It's a useful guide to evaluate if you or other nonaddicted family members could be helped by counseling and/or a support group.

1. Do you worry about how much someone else drinks? Y/N

2. Do you have money problems because of someone else's drinking? Y/N

3. Do you tell lies to cover up for someone else's drinking? Y/N

4. Do you feel that if the drinker loved you, he or she would stop drinking to please you? Y/N

5. Do you blame the drinker's behavior on his or her companions? Y/N

6. Are plans frequently upset or canceled or meals delayed because of the drinker? Y/N

7. Do you make threats, such as, "If you don't stop drinking, I'll leave you"? Y/N

8. Do you secretly try to smell the drinker's breath? Y/N

9. Are you afraid to upset someone for fear it will set off a drinking bout? Y/N

10. Have you been hurt or embarrassed by a drinker's behavior? Y/N

11. Are holidays and gatherings spoiled because of drinking? Y/N

12. Have you considered calling the police for help in fear of abuse? Y/N

13. Do you search for hidden alcohol? Y/N

14. Do you often ride in a car with a driver who has been drinking? Y/N

15. Have you refused social invitations out of fear or anxiety?   Y/N

16. Do you sometimes feel like a failure when you think of the lengths you have gone to control the drinker?   Y/N

17. Do you think that if the drinker stopped drinking, your other problems would be solved?   Y/N

18. Do you ever threaten to hurt yourself to scare the drinker?   Y/N

19. Do you feel angry, confused, or depressed most of the time?   Y/N

20. Do you feel no one understands your problems?   Y/N

If you answered "Yes" to three or more questions, consider counseling, Al-Anon, or some other support group (see Chapter 14 and Resources).

FIRE FIGHTER ARSONISTS

Fire fighter arsonists have been called the fire service's "dirty little secret." The devastation they wreak far exceeds their tiny numbers. Chances are you are reading this chapter not because you know a fire fighter arsonist, but because you or someone you love has been affected by their actions.

The work of fire fighter arsonists has a cascading effect. Not only do they kill and injure people—including fellow fire fighters—and destroy property, they betray the public's trust, damage confidence in the fire service, erode morale, and harm recruitment and fundraising efforts. This in turn influences the quality of affordable training and the purchase of needed equipment. Fire fighter arsonists expose their departments to negative media coverage and increased governmental regulation. And they lay open their coworkers to suspicion, scorn, and ridicule.

It's unthinkable that trained fire fighters—career or volunteer—who are allegedly dedicated to the preservation of life and property, would deliberately set a fire. Who are these people and what motivates them?

Little has been known about fire fighter arsonists until recently. Even today, the information that has been assembled is sketchy. A preliminary profile suggests that the "typical" fire fighter arsonist is a young white male with less than three years of service. He is most often a volunteer. He may be motivated by a need for power and excitement or eager to be a hero—the first to spot the flames, the one to rescue people and property. He may want to test himself, alleviate boredom, practice his skills, collect insurance money, cover a crime, or revenge himself against the department for perceived grievances. He may be part of a group that shows its support for labor actions, such as strikes, by taxing the limits of the replacement forces in an effort to make them look inadequate to the community.

Some fire fighters arsonists are motivated by the wish to make more money. In 2002, an $8.00-an-hour on-call fire fighter set one of the largest wildfires in the history of the state of Arizona. The consequences of his actions in terms of fire suppression and containment reached $10 million, not counting replacement costs for damaged equipment and the loss of personal property. The fire he set destroyed pine forests that took 200 years to mature and created an economic disaster for the local community that depends on the lumber industry for jobs.

Prevention

Firefighter arson is not a trivial problem for the fire service. Its importance is measured not by large numbers of incidents, but by the serious impact of the very few which do occur. . . . The 99.9% of the nation's law-abiding fire and rescue personnel have only to gain from bringing to light the 0.01%. . . . who endanger their colleagues and the citizens they are sworn to protect.
—FIREFIGHTER ARSON: SPECIAL REPORT

Steps are being taken—the most important of which is admitting that there is a problem in the first place. Some of the steps threaten old traditions, particularly in the volunteer sector. While there is no uniform national approach to preventing fire fighter arson, there are some strategies that seem to have worked well on a statewide basis.

Prompt Investigation of Nuisance Fires

Most fire fighter arsonists start with nuisance fires and escalate. They rarely set one fire. (One of the few available studies based on information collected in seven states and one Canadian province found that 66 offenders were responsible for 182 fires.)

There are many reasons to delay reporting suspected fire fighter arson. To start with, most fire fighters and fire chiefs are not trained arson inspectors. Second, it's hard to believe a coworker may be the responsible party. And what are the consequences if you are wrong? Think of the publicity. The influence on morale. The damage to those wrongly accused.

Legal Statutes

The year after South Carolina implemented a law barring anyone with a criminal record from becoming a fire fighter, the number of known fire fighter arson arrests dropped to three from an average of 40 in the previous two years. The law bars any applicant from performing fire fighter duties if he or she has been convicted, pled guilty, pled no contest, or admitted guilt (with or without conviction) to a felony arson-related crime, use of an illegal substance, or abuse of a controlled substance within the last 10 years.

Applicant Screening

Identifying potential arsonists before they are hired or voted in is the best preventive measure. This can be done with a background check that includes a review of the applicant's school, credit, medical history, criminal history, driving, and employment records. There is reason to dig into somebody's school records—many arsonists have a history of juvenile fire setting. According to the FBI, more than 50% of all arson arrests are juveniles. References from previous fire departments and fire service colleagues amend the "official" records and are especially revealing for fire fighters who move from state to state.

Some departments that do not perform background checks require applicants to sign affidavits declaring that they understand the penalties for past or future fire setting. This process appears to discourage applicants with a pattern of troubling past behavior.

Psychological screening and polygraphs fortify the screening process. But they are time-consuming and expensive. As it is, many volunteer departments struggle with instituting even minimal screening procedures for fear of discouraging new applicants.

Education

The "scared straight" approach—educating both seasoned and new fire fighters about the criminal penalties for arson—has shown good results, especially in conjunction with implementing stronger penalties. In addition, these classes are an opportune time to teach fire fighters about fire setting and what to do when they suspect a colleague.

DIVORCE AND INFIDELITY

There's a reporter on the phone asking me if fire fighters have a higher rate of divorce than other occupational groups. She's responding to headlines in the December 1, 2003, *New York Post*: "Bravest Betrayal: Firefighters Leave Wives for Fallen Comrades' 9/11 Widows." I tell her that the U.S. National Center for Health Statistics reports that 50% of *all* first marriages and 60% of *all* remarriages end in divorce. As far as I know, no one tracks divorce statistics by occupation.

Nonetheless, rumors persist. Ask any fire fighter and he or she will declare that the fire service has one of the highest divorce rates in the country. To the contrary, what scant evidence exists suggests just the opposite. It's as though the close bond between fire fighters magnifies and reinforces this dangerous misperception. What's needed is more than rumor control. A distortion like this can mislead couples into thinking that divorce is the inevitable consequence of their normal problems and that getting help is a waste of time and money.

A study of 349 veteran fire fighters in Tulsa, Oklahoma, concluded that 46% of the respondents had been divorced—a bit lower than the national average. But 64% of that same sample still believed fire fighters have a higher divorce rate than the general population. When considering how working in the fire service affected their relationships, 55% of the married fire fighters reported that being a fire fighter had a positive influence on their marriages. Only 24% of those divorced reported that their jobs contributed in any significant way to their divorces.

Other studies of fire fighter and fire fighter/paramedic marriages have found divorce rates ranging from 10 to 32.5%. In one large study, 80% of the married fire fighters reported relatively high rates of satisfaction with the support they received from spouses and family.

One of the few projects to compare employee groups matched fire fighter/EMTs to nonuniform employees working in the same large metropolitan city. The researcher was actually studying the effects of attention deficit disorder on divorce. But when he looked at the frequency of divorce, he found no significant differences between the fire fighter group and the civilian workers.

Infidelity

Getting dependable facts about people's sexual behavior is nearly impossible, even for the most careful researcher. Locker-room talk is hardly a reliable source of information. What seems obvious is that the fire service provides the means and opportunity to be unfaithful. Motive, however, is not so much a consequence of the job as it is a reflection of the people involved: their morals, their maturity, and the lack of satisfaction they have in their ongoing relationships.

Shift work provides plenty of opportunities to be unfaithful. It is also the source of a lot of firehouse humor and urban legend. Several fire fighters told me that they love the 24-hour shift schedule because they know whose wives are home alone and when. And how great it is not to have to pay for a motel room. No surprise that sex talk plays a large part in a youthful, physically fit, action-oriented, male-dominated workforce. And given the way men are conditioned in our society, sex, sometimes illicit sex, offers a distraction—though rarely a solution—for stress, tension, and troubled relationships.

Sometimes the safety net provided by the close-knit fire fighter community becomes tangled. People reach out to comfort one another in hard times. It is not uncommon for divorced or widowed spouses to marry other fire fighters, or for fire fighters to marry their coworkers' friends or relatives, or to work closely with a relative or close friend of an ex-spouse.

Infidelity is a painful experience, but it does not always mean the end of a relationship. It is important to understand the "meaning" the affair has to the people involved. Some marriage experts claim that marriages break up when partners grow apart and no longer feel loved or appreciated. They believe that affairs are less about sex and more about finding an intimate connection: friendship, support, attention, caring, and so on. They encourage couples struggling with infidelity not to "throw in the towel," but to seek help rebuilding what they have lost.

Tips for Dealing with Fire Fighters in Hot Water

- There are a lot of reasons why people get divorced—work may be only one of the primary factors. See Chapter 12 for ideas about when your marriage is in trouble and when you may need outside help.
- If you find yourselves attracted to other people, consider this as a sign that you are lacking something more than sex in your marriage. Acting on the attraction may distract you and give you some temporary satisfaction, but it won't fix what's wrong at home. Talk candidly to your spouse. Seek counseling.
- Never worry more about a person's job than about his or her health. Alcoholism is associated with suicide, domestic violence, brain damage, and premature death. If one of you has a drinking problem, seek help immediately. If the boss finds out, so be it.
- Fire fighters: Build diversity into your life. It's a fallacy that only fire fighters understand other fire fighters. Keep your non–fire fighter friends—you'll benefit from the diversity of activities and perspectives.

- Learn to relax and unwind in a variety of ways that don't involve alcohol.
- Some research indicates that female fire fighters may be more at risk for problem drinking than females in the general population. Monitor yourself—don't assume you are protected because of your gender.
- Take responsibility for monitoring your mental health over time. Alcohol consumption is positively correlated with PTSD, job stress, and years of service for male fire fighters. The more years on the job, the more your exposure to stress and trauma.
- As a public safety family you may have a take-charge, take-action attitude. As a consequence, you may be at risk for doing too much rather than too little for a problem-drinking spouse. Al-Anon recommends stepping back—releasing the alcoholic to make his or her own choices to continue drinking or to stop.
- Alcoholism is a disease that affects the whole family. When any family member changes his or her behavior, it may spur the alcoholic toward recovery more effectively than all the pleading, bargaining, threatening, or arguing you may have tried in the past. But be prepared to feel uncomfortable stepping back—this is uncharted territory. You may feel like you're abandoning your loved one.
- Set a bottom line for what you will and won't tolerate in regard to your loved one's drinking. Once you establish this line, stick to it despite efforts from friends and family to test your resolve.
- Place responsibility where it belongs. Even though alcoholism is a disease, it doesn't absolve the alcoholic from responsibility for his or her choices, including the choice to drink.
- Get your own life back on track. You have issues larger than whether your mate does or doesn't drink. We all need to consider the future, figure out who we are and what we believe in, and find ways to balance our responsibilities to our families, our communities, and ourselves.
- Don't imagine that things will be perfect if and when an alcoholic stops drinking. Recovery from alcoholism is a lifetime commitment with many ups and downs.

CHAPTER **13**

Fire-Fighting Couples

A NEW TRADITION

Fire fighters, both career and volunteer, so love their work that it is common for younger family members to follow in their footsteps. Now that women are serving in the fire service in appreciable numbers, a new family tradition has evolved: the fire fighter couple.

According to a 1995 survey by Women in the Fire Service, 32% of all women fire fighters are married to—or in long-term relationships with—other fire fighters. Nearly three-fourths of these relationships are between fire fighters working in the same department, and most developed after both were hired. This is not an uncommon occurrence. Most of us make enduring relationships at work. When you factor in the intensity of a fire service job—unusual hours, powerful shared experiences, common interests, and a strong emphasis on teamwork—it is easy to see how fire service friendships can lead to romantic involvements. (There are also a growing number of police officer/fire fighter couples. They share some of the advantages that fire fighter couples enjoy and they face some unique challenges generated by the differences in their work cultures.)

There are benefits and dilemmas to being a fire service couple. On the positive side, shift work for professional fire fighters almost guarantees that children will have one parent at home nearly all the time. Fire fighter fathers—providing they don't need to work second jobs—seem to have more time to spend with their kids than do many 9:00–5:00 dads. A dual-career couple—especially one with a third part-time income—may also have more discretionary income than many other families.

Fire fighter couples have a lot in common. They don't have to "translate" for each other or go into long explanations when talking about work. In terms of organizational life, they know all the players and all the challenges. When one has a hard day at work, the other knows exactly what that means.

Fire fighter couples share a sense of humor and a perspective on life that is different from that of most civilians. In particular, they see so much loss and death that they share an appreciation for life as well as a deep understanding of just how fragile life can be.

When things are stressful, they can support each other with feedback, counsel, encouragement, and perspective. They can act as each other's sounding board. They can help in practical ways too—by coaching each other for interviews or studying together for promotional exams. They can work out together and motivate each other to eat well and stay in shape.

But there are dilemmas as well, many of which are similar to those faced by any other dual-career family. Some days fire fighter couples may feel as though they have nothing else in common but their work. Work is all they ever talk about. When things are going badly, they may have a double dose of job stress. They can help each other deal with on-the-job trauma, but sometimes they run the risk of being too close to the incident or the people involved to be of much assistance. And if both are working the same incident, they may each need more than the other has to give.

SOMEONE TO LEAN ON

June is a fire fighter/paramedic and Don is a fire fighter. They met at the fire academy and have been married for five years. Don's the kind of guy who prefers chopping wood to talking about stress. But when June's upset, she wants to vent.

A few years ago June and her partner were deployed to a fire in an encampment of homeless people. Don was there with his truck company. One of the residents had been practicing voodoo and had lit hundreds of candles, creating a flashover that ignited her tent and the surrounding shelters. On the ground next to a stream lay her seven-year-old daughter, barely alive. The child was baked through and covered with fourth-degree burns; her fingers and facial features had burned off. No matter how hard they tried, June and her partner couldn't open an airway in the child's throat.

The details remain crystal-clear in June's memory. The child's family was wailing and throwing themselves on the ground. The sun was setting, the sky was a fiery red, and there were birds screeching in the trees as though they too were in mourning. And then something incredible happened while June was putting the child in the ambulance. She saw the child's "soul" leave her body. "I can't help you," June remembers thinking, "I have to let you go."

At the ER, the on-duty doctor prescribed a shot of morphine. And while he never said it aloud, June understood that he was trying to relieve the child's suffering by hastening her inevitable death.

June was terribly shaken. Never before had she experienced a "vision," though she had heard about other medics who had—they were always mocked and labeled as "nut cases." She couldn't believe this had happened to her—she was tough, hard-boiled, and hadn't a spiritual bone in her body. When Don came into the emergency room, she pulled him into an empty office and started to weep. In her memory, it was the one and only time she ever cried on duty. Don's being there made it safe for her to release her emotions. She wouldn't dare be this self-disclosing in front of anyone else she worked with. But with Don she never has to hide her feelings or explain things. She trusts and confides in him because he is consistently supportive. He never dismisses her feelings or tells her to quit if she can't handle the stress.

COMPETITION

Rick and Sandy are both volunteers. They are active, high-energy people who love excitement. When their pagers go off, they both race to the car eager to drive. The competition is so fierce that they had to create a system to share the driving. They tape a sheet of paper that has been partially torn into strips on the dashboard and write their names on the strips in alternating order: Rick, Sandy, Rick, Sandy, and so on. Whoever drives tears his or her name off so it is clear whose turn it will be next.

Sometimes competitive feelings arise not so much from the partners as from the roles they play in their organization. At first Kitty and Bud had a great deal in common, but after they had their first child they began to worry more about safety and what would happen to their child if they were both hurt on the job. Kitty started studying for promotion and moved into management. That's when their problems started.

Bud is active in a newly formed union seeking increases in salary and benefits. He and Kitty often hold such opposing views on these issues that they have stopped talking about them because it inevitably leads to a fight. The strain is compounded by the fact that both have secrets they cannot share regarding labor negotiations. They are also working different hours: she works 9:00 to 5:00—with a lot of overtime that irritates Bud—and he is on shift: this is both a blessing and a burden.

Occasionally, unhappy fire fighters will complain to Bud about one of Kitty's management decisions instead of going directly to her. Sometimes they accuse her of giving Bud favors. They kid Bud about "sleeping with the enemy" and joke about whether Kitty wears her bars to bed. At parties they don't know whether to treat her like a friend or as a lieutenant. Things are at a stalemate. For the time being they have agreed to disagree in order to avoid pointless fights. Kitty is hoping that Bud will get promoted soon and the gap between them will close.

LIFE IN A FISHBOWL

Bud and Kitty are experiencing a phenomenon common to couples who work together. Their private life is open to comment, criticism, and gossip. It started in the academy when they had to sneak kisses because there was a policy against fraternizing while in uniform. It was particularly painful for Bud to hear the other guys comment on Kitty's physical attributes and speculate about who she was sleeping with. After they married, guys still came up to him with rumors. Bud tries to laugh this stuff off, but he secretly worries; it wouldn't be the first time that two fire fighters had an affair and everyone but the betrayed spouse knew it.

It's understandable that husbands and wives will feel defensive when their mates are criticized, whether personally or professionally. It's particularly hard for men, who may feel especially protective toward their mates, even when their mates are perfectly capable of defending themselves.

That's what happened to Irma and Lamar. Irma is plenty tough—she's been around a long time, well before there were other women in her department. And so, when an eye chart was posted on the department Intranet the day after Irma had an accident driving the rescue truck, she just sloughed it off: "As usual, people are trying to jump in my business and make trouble." But Lamar was furious. Not only was the chart insulting to Irma, the wording—in Ebonics—was racially offensive. "Just because my wife is black they think she can't speak or read proper English," he fumed. Irma didn't share Lamar's outrage and told him he was too thin-skinned; the accident was her fault and she'd take her lumps. But if Lamar wanted to file a complaint he had that right and she wouldn't stop him. After he filed, several people asked Irma to persuade him to change his mind. She held fast. "If you're concerned about it," she said, "ask him yourself."

Lamar and Irma's situation illuminates two very important points that go way beyond who's right and who's wrong. First, fire fighter couples have a unique challenge in remaining true to themselves, to each other, and to their personal and professional futures. Second, it is important for fire fighter couples to maintain their individual identities and resist being seen as a unit.

This is the strategy that Yvonne and James use. James was a fire fighter and Yvonne a nurse when they met and fell in love. James loved his job and his department and Yvonne soon became an active part of his social life. They joined the department's bowling league, participated in charity events, and went to parties. Yvonne felt warmly welcomed by everyone she met. All that abruptly changed when she applied for and was hired as a fire fighter. She was not the first woman hired, but she and James were the first openly declared couple.

Rumors started immediately. Rumor: Yvonne was only hired because the chief owed James a favor. Fact: James scrupulously avoided the chief for fear his relationship with Yvonne would be a deterrent. Rumor: Yvonne cheated on the test because James gave her the answers in advance. Fact: The only assistance James gave her was helping her get in shape and prepping her for the test with flash cards and quiz questions from published study guides.

The early years were terrible, as James knew they would be. There was a lot of fear and resentment toward other female fire fighters in the department and it cascaded down to Yvonne. People Yvonne had previously considered to be friends would leave the room when she entered or avoid looking at her. She was under constant scrutiny. It took two years before she could stop proving she could do the job and three years before she felt socially accepted. It was the hardest time of her life. What kept her going was her own dogged persistence and James's belief that she had what it took to do the job justice and the potential to be a role model for women in the fire service. Whenever she felt at the end of her rope, James helped her stay focused. His knowledge and perspective on department dynamics was a blessing.

From the outset they made a conscious and deliberate effort to present themselves as individuals. Yvonne kept her maiden name. While it hurt to hear some of the comments made about women in the fire service, James never allowed himself to be baited into a fight. He was clear about his position on women fire fighters, but he never fell into the trap of taking things personally or responding to rumors about what people were saying about Yvonne.

At home it was a slightly different story. Yvonne needed to talk about what was happening at work, but she worried about how much to share because she didn't want to damage James's relationships with his friends. Whenever he asked Yvonne if she wanted him to talk to someone or straighten things out, she always refused, saying she had to handle her own problems. In fact, she now gets along well with some folks James doesn't like and vice versa. They make up their own minds about people and try not to let the other's experience be an undue influence. And while

James finds it hard to forgive and forget some of the rude things that were done or said, he hasn't let it derail him: after all that has happened he still loves his job and his department.

Five years later, they continue to use this strategy. Whenever someone asks Yvonne what James thinks about something, she tells them to ask him. When the company officer (CO) calls James to inquire if either he or Yvonne are available for overtime, James tells the CO to telephone Yvonne directly. They never speak for each other, make commitments for each other, or volunteer for each other. They try never to work at the same station. But even when circumstances force one to ship out to the other's station, they have become so good at "disconnecting" on the job that the new people don't even know they're married.

THE SECOND SHIFT: ON DUTY AT HOME

I'm talking to Ricky and Stan. They are a very happy couple, married nine years, who think fire fighter marriages give both partners the best of all possible worlds: an exciting job and lots of family time. When Ricky and I are alone I ask her how they have managed domestic chores and childcare for their three kids. She tells me that they have traditional roles. She cares for the kids most of the time, washes clothes, and cleans house while he pays the bills, does yard work, and maintains their cars. They share childrearing but she is still the primary caregiver and disciplinarian. "Oh well," she sighs, "that's just life."

Later on when I'm talking to Stan alone he answers the same question in a different way. In terms of chores, they each do what they do best. He handles things outside the house and she handles things inside the house, although they switch roles as necessity dictates. "Sometimes," he says, "I do the wash and Ricky mows the lawn."

Before they had children, Stan and Ricky both had side jobs they loved. Since the children were born, Ricky has cut her hours back to almost nothing. Stan has not. Ricky arranges all childcare. When she goes somewhere without Stan she leaves behind a packed diaper bag and prepares all the meals. It's not that he doesn't care about his children—he adores them and plays with them hours on end. But, according to Ricky, she's the "organized" one and he's the "spontaneous" one. Most of the thinking and planning falls to her. She knows several other fire fighter couples in their very large department and Ricky says their dynamics are similar: the women shoulder more than half the domestic responsibilities. This is how men and women are raised in our culture. Being a fire fighter couple doesn't override that.

HAVING CHILDREN

Forty-three percent of fire fighter couples have children at home. Like Kitty and Bud, having children makes fire fighter couples more aware of the dangers they face and the consequences to their children. This can prompt them to make unanticipated career choices.

Some women, like Kitty, have a difficult time getting back into good physical condition within the time allotted for maternity leave, which affects their self-confidence and self-esteem. Staying in shape—a challenge for everyone—may become more difficult with age and repeated pregnancies.

Catching up on your sleep when you have children is also a challenge—one made easier when your spouse understands why you're so tired. I have a telephone appointment with Walt and Amy on a beautiful, sunny Saturday afternoon. Walt answers the phone. Amy is asleep and he is minding the children, who start to cry the minute he begins to talk. "Amy caught a two-alarm fire last night," Walt tells me, "and she needs to sleep." He's neither angry nor irritated that their plans to go boating have changed. "Who knows," he says, "maybe tomorrow I'll pull an all-nighter and come home exhausted."

Happy fire fighter couples learn to respect each other's sleep patterns. Walt and Amy are like the Hare and the Turtle. He has seemingly endless energy and races around all day until he falls into bed, at which point Amy can't rouse him no matter how hard she tries. Amy, on the other hand, is a light sleeper who restores her energy by napping during the day. If she can't grab "40 winks," meaning a 10-minute minisleep, she is groggy and grumpy. There is no normal pattern. Everyone is wired differently.

Childcare

By far, the biggest challenge facing fire fighter couples (and single parents) is childcare. Couples who work the same shift and have the same days off need to find reliable 24-hour childcare—a scarce commodity. Couples who work different shifts seldom need a baby-sitter, but they hardly see each other and can wind up feeling like single parents with two incomes. Many of the couples I interviewed said their lives would be impossible without the help of relatives or a reliable baby-sitter who functions as a "third grandmother."

With the increase in fire fighter couples comes an increased need for dependable 24-hour childcare facilities that offer flexible care options to accommodate early morning shift changes, large-scale emergencies, wildfires, off-duty recalls, and other events that ordinary childcare providers don't cover. There are a few departments in the United States and Britain that offer on-site, round-the-clock care or subsidies for off-site childcare, but these are rare indeed.

THE OTHER WOMAN

M. J. prefers to socialize with other fire fighter couples, because, to quote her, "Other women don't get me." M. J. and her husband, Pete, work in a very large urban fire department that employs many women and has a dozen or more fire fighter couples—too many to count. Even still it's new territory for many non–fire fighter wives; they feel threatened by the presence of women in the firehouse and they don't hide it.

M. J. was prepared for this. Her uncle was a fire fighter and she observed how uncomfortable her aunt and her aunt's friends were when women were first hired. Their initial reaction was fear that women would compromise their husbands' safety; their second reaction was jealousy. While apprehensions have eased considerably with younger families who are accustomed to seeing men and women work side by side—though not sleep side by side—they haven't entirely gone away.

M. J. and Pete went to a party thrown by some of Pete's firehouse friends. M. J. got all dressed up, something she rarely does. It was a pleasure to get out of her uniform and her sweats—which is what she wears most of the time—and to put on high heels and a slinky dress. She hardly ever gets the chance to feel feminine or sexy these days. When Pete was introducing her around, some of his buddies' wives were impressed that a petite, feminine woman had what it took to be a fire fighter. Others were standoffish and some were downright rude. "How did *you* make it through fire school?", one wife asked, implying that M. J. must have slept her way to graduation. One woman warned her to "stay away from my husband"—a man who was so overweight and old, by M. J.'s standards—that M. J. was stunned. "Yes, Ma'am," she replied, "but I want you to know that I have a husband of my own—I don't need another one." At that the other woman laughed, relaxed visibly, and seemed friendlier.

M. J. thinks that women like this must have shaky marriages. She concedes that in her department there have been some extramarital relationships between older fire fighters and young, female rookies that have led to divorce and remarriage. This prompts her to take the precautionary step of explaining to wives she has just met—as soon as the conversation permits—that she and Pete met in the academy. She does not want to be mistaken for a "husband stealer."

In the station house visiting wives sometimes keep their distance and treat her and the other women fire fighters with coolness; they don't make eye contact, they ignore them, and they don't respond to greetings. On the phone, wives will demand to know who she is, especially when she has shipped out to a station where women don't usually work. M. J.'s strategy is to "kill 'em with kindness." She tries not to take things personally and rarely gets defensive or overreacts.

Tips for Fire Fighter Couples

- Keep your non–fire fighter friends: they'll bring variety and fresh perspective into your lives and keep you from becoming isolated.
- Sharing your love of the job is not enough to make a marriage work. What happens if one of you is injured and has to leave the service? Diversify your outside interests and develop new ones you hold in common. Having a variety of activities or hobbies makes you more intriguing to each other. Shop-talk gets boring faster than you think.
- Work at different stations. If you spend too much time together at work, you risk not having enough to talk about at home and you may find yourselves going your separate ways off duty.
- Keep your personal affairs private—to do otherwise is to risk falling into the rumor mill. It's a sign of marital distress when you find yourselves confiding in other people about relationship difficulties instead of talking to each other. It's comforting and helpful to talk with friends and family, but it doesn't solve the problem you're having at home.
- Balance career goals with family goals. Be realistic about how much children will change your lives. Discuss in advance how you will share domestic responsibilities. Take into consideration your agency's maternity and parental leave policies and the opportunities for job sharing or part-time work.
- Have an emergency childcare plan for your family. In a big incident you may both be working. Join or form a baby-sitting cooperative. Baby-sit for your friends and neighbors whenever possible; you may need to call in your "IOUs" in an emergency.
- Don't let others think that you can't or won't compete against one another or that the more important opportunities should automatically go to the male partner first. You will need to make adjustments for each other's career, but if either of you sacrifices too much, you risk feeling resentful.
- Don't let anyone else assume that being parents—especially being a mother—puts you out of the running for tough assignments.

- Develop support systems outside of your family. Because you love someone doesn't mean you automatically understand each other or know how best to provide support. In the unlikely event that you are both involved in the same critical incident, you may each need more than the other has to give.
- Fire fighters are problem solvers, rescuers, fixers, and natural-born helpers. Use these skills tactfully at home, especially when it comes to giving feedback about work performance. Always ask your mate if he or she wants your advice or feedback. Women frequently complain that their husbands are too quick with advice when all they want is someone to listen to them. On the other hand, marital experts claim that males are not sufficiently open to their wives' influence.
- Insist that people at work treat you as individuals, not as an inseparable unit. Be your own person. Fight your own battles, claim your own achievements.
- Keep your personal issues at home: no one wants to be around a couple who are quarreling or romancing at work. No one wants to go through one employee to reach another or to debate orders with a worker's spouse.

CHAPTER **14**

Getting Help

Jon Carroll, a columnist for the *San Francisco Chronicle*, wrote a humorous advice column for men wanting to meet women. "The best way," he said, " . . . is to stand on a busy corner in any large city. Eventually someone will ask you for directions. That person is a woman."

His technique for distinguishing men from women arises from a popular stereotype that men are reluctant to ask for directions when lost. That same stereotype further characterizes men as wary about sharing vulnerable feelings and unwilling to seek needed professional help. Sad to say, this is not just hackneyed typecasting. Studies consistently support the stereotype: men *are* less likely than women to recognize emotional problems or to seek formal and informal help for their distress.

If you're a woman reading this chapter, the probability is that you recognize that something is bothering you or someone you love. Perhaps you are the person who feels most responsible for change when things aren't going well in your family or in your relationships. Maybe you're the one most in need of things to change.

WHY DO PEOPLE NEED COUNSELING?

There are lots of reasons people want professional help. Some people are deeply disturbed and their lives are unbearable. Other people are interested in personal growth; they may be slightly unhappy or feeling that they're just not living up to their potential. Still others have a specific issue—a decision or a dilemma—that they want to discuss with a neutral third party. One thing is certain: you don't have to be crazy to seek therapy. In fact, most therapy clients fall into a category I call the "worried well." They have a problem to solve and will solve it, usually in a few sessions.

Here is a partial list of the reasons people enter counseling:

- Emotional pain
- Poor self-esteem
- Difficulties coping with daily life
- Difficulties coping with work
- High stress and/or stress-related medical problems
- Depression—from low grade to severe in degree
- Worries, anxieties, fears, phobias, and panic attacks
- Posttraumatic stress reactions
- Marital and sexual problems
- Relationship problems with friends, family, spouses, or co-workers
- Career concerns
- Grief
- Addiction to drugs, alcohol, gambling, eating, smoking, or spending
- Big decisions to make
- Behavioral problems
- Nightmares, trouble sleeping
- Feeling stuck
- Feeling suicidal

CHOOSING A THERAPIST

There is a bewildering array of legitimate mental health professionals from which to choose. Be aware that anyone can hang out a shingle and call him- or herself a psychotherapist. When you pick a therapist, make sure that person is licensed or properly registered. Licensure and registration don't guarantee a successful outcome, but they do indicate that your therapist has met minimum requirements in terms of training and supervision, carries malpractice insurance, and is bound by professional ethics. Don't be afraid to ask about confidentiality, fees, office policies, expected length of treatment, theoretical considerations, or the "state of the art" therapy for your problem—whatever is on your mind. If the therapist doesn't want to discuss your concerns or won't give you a satisfactory answer, move on.

Most competent therapists will give new patients a written copy of their office policies regarding payment, billing, sliding-scale fees, and limits of confidentiality. They will also ask you to complete a health history and sign several forms—for example, a consent-to-treatment agreement, and statements indicating that you have received and read copies of your rights of privacy, your rights as a patient, and how to file a complaint.

There are several main categories of mental health professionals and a whole lot of newly minted, sometimes questionable, classifications. Among the main categories are psychiatrists (MDs), who are medical doctors with specialized training in psychiatry or neuropsychiatry. They are the people to consult about medication and physical conditions affecting someone's mental state. Your internist can also prescribe psychotropic medication—you may want to begin by consulting him or her. (By the time this book is published, psychologists in some states may also be licensed to prescribe psychotropic medication.) Clinical psychologists (with a PhD or PsyD) have doctorate degrees and specialize in treating emotional or behavioral problems and conducting psychological assessments. Clinical social workers (with a MSW or a LCSW) have master's degrees and take a social systems approach to treating individuals and families. Other master's-level therapists (with a MA or a MS) may have graduate degrees in psychology, clinical counseling, marriage and family counseling, or a specialized field such as psychiatric nursing, addiction, health, or grief counseling.

Some of these academic distinctions are irrelevant. What counts most is compassion, availability, integrity, and "good chemistry" between the therapist and the client. There are exceptions, of course, but, generally speaking, public safety personnel feel most comfortable with plain-speaking, practical, down-to-earth therapists who know the fire fighter culture and aren't afraid to interact actively, use appropriate humor, answer questions, and make suggestions.

Bernie called his employee assistance program (EAP) for bereavement counseling four months after his father died. He wasn't sleeping well and he felt overwhelmed with responsibility for his mother, who was "falling apart." He was also consumed with guilt. As a fire fighter/paramedic, he had many "saves" to his credit, but he couldn't save his father from the pain and misery of a long and wasting death. Asking for help wasn't easy. He got an appointment with a counselor right away, but he thought the therapist was a little strange because she barely said anything and Bernie felt like he was floundering. He'd never seen a "shrink" before and he didn't know where to start or what to say. When he finally "opened up," it was well into the hour, at which point the therapist "abruptly" ended the session. Bernie was so hurt and angry he never returned. "What for?", he asked, "the guys at the firehouse are that good to me."

It's hard to know what really happened. Maybe the therapist was incompetent or insensitive. Maybe she was inexperienced—some EAPs pay a minimum fee, meaning that they contract primarily with young professionals who are just beginning to build a practice. Maybe Bernie didn't give her a chance. Therapists can't read minds or work miracles. They need enough time to get to know you, your problems, and your style. Therapy isn't a "load and go" operation; you can't expect any therapist to react as swiftly and decisively as you do on your job.

Buyer Beware I

Public safety personnel generally have good instincts about people. On the other hand, especially in times of stress, people can overvalue education and authority and undervalue their own gut hunches about someone. That's why it's important to know that while there is wide variety in therapeutic practice, there are some things that are simply unacceptable.

Good therapists value *your* time as much as their *own*. They don't break appointments at the last minute or fail to show up. If they do, they have a good reason and are willing to discuss your feelings about it and perhaps offer you a free session. They don't fall asleep during therapy sessions or routinely take nonemergency phone calls. They are properly dressed and their offices, even home offices, are professionally furnished and their licenses are on display.

Competent therapists keep clear boundaries between themselves and their clients. They do not flirt, touch their clients improperly, solicit or engage in sexual activity, ask for dates, or suggest socializing away from the consulting room. And they don't barter or exchange goods or employment for therapy.

Conscientious therapists are open about their treatment plans and diagnoses. They take a collaborative approach and will never force you to do anything that feels uncomfortable. They respect your boundaries and know that you have a right to refuse any type of treatment or to end treatment without obligation or harassment.

Where to Look for a Therapist

Large career departments often have in-house counseling programs where mental health professionals work directly for the department and have offices onsite or in a separate building. Because they interact with the workforce in other capacities such as training, they know the day-to-day dynamics of the department. On the other hand, their immersion in the organization may cause fire fighters to worry about trusting them with confidential information.

Other departments contract with external EAPs or managed care agencies whose job it is to refer you to the practitioner who best meets your needs in terms of specialty, location, and any other preferences you may have. If you don't like the first one you meet, he or she should give you another referral. These outside providers have a firmer "fire wall" between themselves and the department, but, as mentioned above, they may be inexperienced therapists or therapists who don't know the fire service culture.

Check your medical insurance for mental health benefits. Many plans cover a set number of outpatient sessions or treatments for substance abuse. Often these sessions must first be authorized by your primary care physician.

Other sources for counseling or referrals are family service agencies, the Red Cross, and your state or county mental health associations. If you live near a college, university, or private school of psychology, check to see if they have a counseling clinic. Such clinics are staffed by interns, some of whom may be experienced midcareer professionals. All interns receive weekly supervision, so you get the benefit of two mental health professionals for the price of one.

Don't forget to ask your friends. One of the best ways to find a therapist is to get a name from someone who has been in therapy, feels good about the experience, and has had positive results.

Peer Supporters and Chaplains

Peer supporters and chaplains are the supportive backbone of many fire departments. Peer supporters have walked in your shoes—they understand what you're going through because they probably have been through it themselves. Many but not all have been trained to listen, help you to help yourself, and refer you to competent mental health assistance if you need it.

Likewise, fire department chaplains are there to offer nondenominational spiritual guidance to fire fighters and victims. They are dedicated individuals who seem to be available at any time of the day or night. While some have training in psychology or critical incident stress, their expertise is pastoral, not psychological. Select a peer supporter or a chaplain with the same care that you use to select a therapist.

Self-Help Groups

There seems to be no substitute for the authentic compassion and empathy that comes from talking with others who share your experiences and problems. There are literally thousand of self-help groups. Some have a long history, like Alcoholics Anonymous (AA); others, like the victim's groups formed after 9/11, are born out of recent necessity. Some groups are primarily supportive and others also advocate for causes related to the group's mission (see Resources).

Use care when selecting a self-help group. Avoid groups that encourage feeling victimized or that promote a "poor me" philosophy. Be especially wary of groups that discourage you from consulting anyone outside the group or make it hard for you to leave. Self-help groups work well in tandem with professional counseling. Each can optimize the benefits of the other.

What Will It Cost?

In-house programs are usually free. EAPS and managed care generally require a copayment that varies depending on the contract negotiated. The cost is usually not prohibitive. Private therapy is expensive, and fees vary according to where you live. Private therapists may have sliding-scale fees for financially strapped new clients or reserve some spots for ongoing clients who have financial emergencies. Family service agencies, state and county facilities, universities, and other subsidized clinics generally offer low-cost or sliding-scale fees for qualifying clients. Expect to have to document your eligibility. Peer support, chaplains' programs, and self-help groups are free.

CONFIDENTIALITY

Licensed and certified mental health professionals are required by statute and by their professional codes of ethics to keep all patient records confidential. If they fail to do this, they risk losing their licenses, their livelihoods, and exposing themselves to lawsuits. (Recent federal legislation known as the Health Insurance Portability and Accountability Act [HIPPA] has fortified patient confidentiality even further.)

Therapists sometimes seem to care more about confidentiality than their clients do. A fire chief had his secretary enter his therapy appointments on a computerized office calendar—the same calendar that was available to everyone in his management group. The office gossip that ensued obviously didn't come from his therapist. Another fire fighter told his wife that he was seeing the department psychologist, but neglected to tell her why. His wife assumed he was unhappy with her and called the therapist in a panic. The therapist was sympathetic, but unwilling to talk to her or even to acknowledge that her husband was in treatment.

Therapists are fierce guardians of their clients' privileged communication because they know that psychotherapy only works in an atmosphere of trust and safety. When that trust is broken, it has a chilling effect on clients and potential clients everywhere.

There are, however, limits to confidentiality. The following are circumstances in which a therapist is permitted or obliged to break confidentiality and is not held liable for doing so.

• If you are a threat to yourself or others, your therapist has a duty to warn your intended victim(s) and to inform the police. Therapists do not take this duty lightly; they won't break confidentiality on the basis of a off-hand remark such as "I'm so mad at my captain I could kill him." But expect to be asked about this in detail; your therapist will be trying to determine how serious you are (see section on suicide, below).

• If you are physically, emotionally, or sexually abusing a child or an elderly person, your therapist must report it to the police or to the appropriate protective agency. The same holds true when a child or elderly victim reveals current or prior abuse.

• If you are so gravely disabled that you are unable to care for yourself, your therapist must report this.

• Good therapists seek supervision and consultation about difficult cases, and they are required to get ongoing training. Under these circumstances, they may present "cases," but without names or identifying details. This is not careless cocktail-party gossip—it is how therapists enhance their skills.

• In most states, if you file a lawsuit claiming damage to your mental health you waive confidentiality for past or present mental health treatment. The same holds true when you file a workers' compensation claim because the treating therapist is required to submit monthly reports about your progress and your prognosis.

• Insurance carriers require therapists to provide patient information for billing purposes. This information is usually restricted to dates of sessions, services provided, diagnosis, prognosis, and the therapist's fees. You will be asked to sign a release-of-information form when you enroll in your plan.

Managed health care organizations and EAPs may require additional detailed information if your therapist requests more than your allotted sessions. These details are not shared with your employer. What your employer receives are utilization reports. For example, the employer may get a summary showing how many employees applied for counseling services, how many sessions they used, what departments they work in (fire, police, public works, etc.), and into what categories their major concerns fell:

work, family, eldercare, financial problems, smoking cessation, and so on. They never get names.

• You have no confidentiality if you are mandated to attend counseling or to be evaluated as fit for duty. In these cases, you are not the client, your employer is. In the case of mandated counseling, the information your employer can obtain is usually limited to whether you missed any appointments and what might assist you in the workplace. It's always better to seek counseling yourself before being ordered to go to counseling. But if you are mandated, you can still get something out of it, including an opportunity to save your job.

Fitness-for-duty evaluations are thorough psychological investigations involving hours of clinical interviews, objective psychological tests, an extensive review of your work and personal history, and third-party collateral interviews, as necessary. The information they generate should be extensive—after all, your job is on the line. Even so, the final report delivered to your employer is limited to the following: (1) enough information to document the presence or absence of job-related psychological problems that can be expected to interfere with your ability to do your job, and (2) a clear opinion that you are permanently or temporarily fit (with or without accommodations) or unfit. Details of your past and present life should not be included in the report.

Mandatory counseling and fitness-for-duty evaluations are used far less in the fire service than they are in law enforcement. Lack of experience or the absence of standardized procedures can make the process more awkward and uncomfortable than it already is. Fitness-for-duty evaluations are appropriate when an employee engages in observable, problematic, job-related behavior. They should never be used as punishment or as a substitute for competent supervision.

• You have no confidentiality when talking to peer supporters or attending critical incident group debriefings—even those conducted by licensed mental health professionals—because no one can guarantee that all members of the group will keep what is said to themselves. A few states protect the confidentiality of your conversations with peer supporters, but most do not. This doesn't mean you should avoid talking to peer supporters, but you should recognize that there are some things that you may not want to disclose.

Buyer Beware II

Therapy is not a feel-good experience, it is about change. New clients in my office sign a consent-to-treatment form that says "Participating in therapy can be beneficial in many ways beyond the resolution of those specific concerns that led you to seek therapy. Working toward these benefits, however, requires effort and may create some discomfort." It's a paradox: sometimes you have to feel badly in the service of feeling better or you have to lose control in order to get it back.

Some people enter therapy with what I call "a 15-year overnight problem." A lot of the pain of therapy comes from facing what they've been avoiding. The loss of control comes from expressing stifled emotions. People who don't allow themselves to cry, for example, are often irrationally afraid that when they finally open the floodgates they'll never be able to stop.

There are surprises in therapy and frustrations too. You may seek counseling for one problem and wind up working on another one. You may bring your spouse in for help and discover that you are the one causing the trouble or at least making an equal contribution. Coming to therapy to change someone else doesn't work. It's hard enough to change yourself—just think of the last time you attempted to diet or start an exercise program.

To be successful in therapy, your goals must be achievable, manageable, and supportable. That means you won't be perfect as a result of counseling, but you will probably be more accepting of your own imperfect self. You and your counselor should talk about your goals early in the process.

Therapy is a team effort. Fire fighters are used to working in teams. Your therapist is only as good as the information you share. Be as open as possible. Eva came to counseling for help adjusting to being the only female in her department. Her therapist seemed fixed on getting her to quit or apply somewhere else, while Eva was determined to hang in there. It was very frustrating and it felt as though they were working at cross-purposes. When

Eva brought this up to the therapist, they were able to work it out. Sometimes you have to help your therapist to help you.

WHEN TO GO

The best advice is to get help sooner rather than later. When a fire department thinks about calling out the strike team, they don't wait long before making the final decision. Better to assemble the team and dismiss it than to not have it ready when needed.

The same principle applies to personal counseling. I know that self-reliant people like fire fighters and their families want to first try solving their own problems. And it's true that talking to friends, family, peers, and religious advisors helps, as does the passage of time. So if you're thinking about consulting a professional, it may mean that you've done what you can on your own and you're telling yourself it's now time to do something more. Admitting you need help is a hard first step, one that takes guts. Most fire fighters would rather run into a burning building than sit down in a therapist's office.

Code 2 Calls: Couple and Family Therapy

A Code 2 response in the fire service means get to the scene safely and swiftly, without exceeding the speed limit and without turning on the lights and siren. How people define "swift" in their personal lives varies. According to some studies, couples with marriage problems wait six years from the time trouble strikes until they seek professional assistance. That's much too long. By the time these couples get to counseling, they're fighting more and feeling further alienated from each other. Pity the poor therapist: instead of having a brush fire to quell, the entire forest is ablaze.

How do you know when your marriage or your relationship is in trouble? While each couple and each family is different, there are a few rules of thumb, some of which have been developed by Dr. John Gottman, marital researcher and therapist. Dr. Gottman studied 3,000 couples over a period of 30 years in an effort to predict which relationships would end in divorce. Essentially he found that troubled relationships are characterized by a preponderance of negativity while happy marriages had a 5:1 ratio of positive interactions. Dr. Gottman's findings have filled several books and can't be summarized here. But you can go to his website and complete the relationship quizzes. Use your results to determine if you and your spouse could profit from counseling (see Resources).

Code 3 Calls: Suicide and Domestic Abuse

Code 3 calls are a step up. They indicate the situation is urgent and fire personnel need to get there in a hurry—with lights on and sirens blaring. Similar urgency is required for suicidal behavior and domestic abuse because there is danger involved.

While neither suicide nor domestic abuse is known to be widespread in the fire service, the subjects are too important to ignore for the few families that may need help. The brief information included here is meant to guide the reader toward help and encourage you to use the Resources listed at the end of the book.

Suicide

Most people who commit suicide give hints—some clear, some coded—that they are thinking of killing themselves or that they are deeply distressed about something. Occasionally people will kill themselves with absolutely no warning. In either case, the legacy of suicide is powerful and enduring, leaving the survivors with questions and emotions that may persist for decades and influence generations to come.

People commit suicide for a variety of reasons, some known only to themselves:

- Depression or other emotional illnesses (see below).
- Altruism: The belief that others will be better off without them.
- Hopelessness and helplessness: Suicide seems to be the best and only solution to their problems.
- Revenge: Others will be sad or sorry for how they acted.

- Impulsive rage: Anger at self or others, often fueled by alcohol.
- Significant loss: The desire to reunite with a dead spouse, child, or friend—sometimes on the anniversary of their deaths or births.
- Potential loss: Real or imagined fear of losing a job or a relationship.
- Shame: The severest form of self-criticism.

Warning Signs for Suicide. Any of the above mindsets is cause for concern and a call to seek professional assistance. Depression, especially short-term stress-related depression, can often be successfully treated with psychotherapy, medication, hospitalization, or a combination of all three. Don't be afraid to confront your loved one with your concerns. Intervention is the key to preventing suicide. The consequences of getting help are never as permanent as the consequences of suicide.

No one has a crystal ball. Even seasoned mental health experts can miss the signs. Public safety personnel are adept at "sucking it up," masking their internal distress. But there are a few red flags that indicate that the potential for self-harm is great and prompt professional intervention is required. It is especially worrisome and dangerous when the following indicators pile up. One of the deadliest pileups may be when substance abuse and the real or potential loss of a relationship combine with problems at work.

- *Depression.* Serious depression is more than a case of the blues. Depressed people have a sad, hopeless, negative outlook on life. They may be lethargic and slow moving or irritable, restless, and bitter. They might have trouble sleeping (or sleep too much) and lack appetite or sex drive. Their appearance or hygiene may decline. They lose their sense of humor and take little interest or pleasure in social activities. They seem distracted and different from their usual selves. And they feel this way nearly every day, all day, for a minimum of two weeks. (Note: any major change in personality is cause for concern and may signal psychological or physical illness.)
- *Preoccupation with suicide.* When someone frequently reads

and talks about other people killing themselves, this should merit your attention—especially if they appear comfortable with the idea of suicide, express admiration for people who take their own lives, and openly declare that death is preferable to life or life is not worth living.

• *Suicide threats and attempts.* It is a myth that people who threaten to kill themselves or make abortive attempts are not truly serious. Do not try to decipher their real intentions by yourself: consult a professional.

• *A burst of joy following a suicidal crisis.* Someone who displays a surge of happiness or energy within months following a suicidal crisis is a cause for concern. The person may have decided to commit suicide and what he or she is feeling is relief to have finally come to this conclusion. These deaths are exceptionally shocking because friends and family have been deceived into thinking their loved one was getting better.

• *Increased substance abuse.* Because alcohol and drugs lower inhibitions, they are frequently associated with suicide. Furthermore, alcohol and other drugs amplify the risk factors for suicide because they act as depressants, increase paranoia, and create behavioral problems that can lead to personal and professional ruin.

• *Tangible preparations.* Things are dire indeed when a person has the means to kill him- or herself and has already made a plan. The more specific and detailed the plan, the more desperate and imminent the need to get this person to a safe place where help is available.

• *Giving things away and reckless behavior.* When people break off relationships and/or give away their valued possessions, this may be a sign they have decided to die. The same is true for reckless behavior. When a usually careful fire fighter starts taking chances—freelancing, not wearing SCBA, driving while drunk— he may be hoping to disguise his suicide as an accident or to die as a hero.

Domestic Abuse

Domestic abuse is a serious problem in the United States. Experts claim that 20–30% of married couples will experience violence at some point in their relationships. Every year two to four million women and 100,000 men are victims of domestic violence and three to ten million children are at risk for witnessing it. Children who witness abuse at home suffer psychological problems that can extend into adulthood and affect their future families. Witnessing violence may not be all that befalls them; a high percentage of men who batter women also batter their children.

Experts in the field say that people who suffer from PTSD, substance abuse, or mental illness may have a tendency toward domestic abuse. None of these conditions excuse violence; all are a reason to seek treatment.

Disintegrating families are at great peril. Couples who are divorcing, separated, or living apart report three times more severe violence than do intact families. Women who choose to leave abusive partners remain at considerable risk.

Violence is only the tip of the iceberg. There is a whole range of abusive and controlling behaviors that may persist before physical violence erupts. Abusers are verbally insulting, humiliating, and intimidating. They control their victims by isolating them from friends and family, restricting their movements, and limiting their access to money. They insist on rigid gender roles. They may threaten to hurt children, pets, even themselves to get their way. They rarely if ever take responsibility for their actions. Instead, they minimize their behavior and/or blame their victims for causing it.

Make no mistake about it: domestic abuse is not about anger or disagreement. Most couples get angry and fight. Partner abuse occurs when one partner uses anger or force to dominate the other and to control his or her behavior. Don't fool yourself into thinking that you're safe because your relationship has not yet become violent or your spouse seems truly remorseful for his actions. This is a typical pattern. Without intervention, these periods of regret and kindness will get shorter as the pushing, shoving, glaring, yelling, or smashing things escalates into far more dangerous actions like punching, choking, or worse.

Ask yourself: Am I afraid of my mate? If you answer "Yes," get help immediately, but go alone to begin with. Couple counseling can exacerbate the abuse.

Tips for Dealing with Suicidal Behavior

- If someone you know commits suicide, get help for yourself. You will be full of questions, anger, and self-blame. Remember that people who kill themselves are responsible for their choices. If they are determined, nothing or no one can stop them.
- Be direct with suicidal people. Avoid using euphemisms—don't be afraid to use the words "suicide" and "killing yourself." You can't put the idea in someone's head if it isn't already there.
- Avoid cheering people up—it doesn't work and it feels hollow. But do give hope. Hope is the awareness of options or the memory of having survived tough times.
- Empathize with the person's pain but point out there may be less drastic ways to end it. Try to understand how and why the suicidal individual has arrived at this point. Never lecture or sermonize.
- Offer to support this person getting help—make the appointment, drive him or her to the doctor's office. But only make offers you can reasonably support. The consequences of letting this person down are too great for both of you.

Tips for Dealing with Domestic Abuse

- Keep your standards high right from the beginning. Do not tolerate verbal, emotional, or physical abuse or any kind of hurtful behavior.
- If you need help, call your local domestic abuse hotline or the toll-free national hotline at 800.799.SAFE. They will provide support, information, and assistance making a safety plan.
- Find a therapist who specializes in domestic abuse. Avoid counselors who seem to have their own agendas. It is up to you to decide if you leave or stay.
- Safety for yourself and your children is your top priority. Only you can decide how safe it is to fight back.

Epilogue

Shortly before my brother, Richard, retired as a volunteer fire fighter, he was eating in a restaurant with some friends. As the waiter served his companions, the chef appeared from the kitchen dressed in his traditional white coat and tall hat. He was carrying a plate piled high with food and he set it down in front of my brother.

"I guess you don't remember me," the chef said. "I was in a terrible car wreck. When you got there I was lying on the ground and while we waited for the paramedics you held my hand and re-assured me I would be fine. It made all the difference in the world to me and I wanted to thank you."

My brother was astonished. He had no idea how the chef recognized him and he, in turn, could hardly believe that the healthy man who stood in front of him was the same frightened victim he remembered lying on the ground covered with dirt and blood, with a cannula in his nose and a cervical collar on his neck. It was an amazing reunion and the memory of it will stay with my brother for the rest of his life.

Making a significant difference in someone's life is a pleasure reserved for very few people. Fire fighters and their families are among this elite group; you can take pride in the fact that some-how people are alive because of you, somewhere houses are standing because of you, and most times people sleep better be-cause of you.

There is no doubt about the value of the services fire fighters perform in their communities or the rewards that accrue from doing such challenging work. It's gratifying to know what to do in a crisis and to be able to act when others hold back. Fire fighters and their families have chosen to be part of something bigger than themselves. As a result, they are privileged to witness and participate in life's most intense moments. The curtain between what is public and what is private parts when fire fighters appear. In a world that sometimes seems superficial and materialistic, their work is real, genuine, and intimate.

Today, as I was driving home from my office, I was forced to turn off the road because of a multivehicle accident. I pulled over and watched as police officers, fire fighters, and fire fighter/paramedics went about their work, each an integral and necessary part of a long chain of emergency responders that includes at one end the dispatcher who answered the 911 call and at the other end the ER team of doctors, nurses, and technicians.

Fire fighters' families are the unacknowledged and often invisible links in this chain. It is your steadfast support that releases fire fighters to work on behalf of others and welcomes them home again, no matter what kind of day they've had. Fire fighters and their families assume risks so that others can feel secure. Please, take as good care of yourselves as you do the rest of us.

Resources

This list of organizations, websites, books, reports, and people may be useful in times of trouble. I have relied on some of these resources for years, others are new to me. In no case should any listing be taken as an endorsement.

I classified the resources into topical sections for easier searching. There is some overlap and you may have to look in more than one section for a relevant resource. The sections are listed alphabetically: alcohol and drug abuse; diversity; domestic violence; family matters; health and safety; line-of-duty deaths; mental health and psychological support; organizational stress; referral and treatment; stress management; suicide; and volunteers.

As I created this list of resources, I found that those targeted to fire fighter families were a drop in a veritable sea of resources for fire fighters. It is my hope that this list will expand in time, and that fire fighter families will reach out to each other, make connections, get support, share ideas, and build resources for the future.

ALCOHOL AND DRUG ABUSE

Organizations and Websites

Alcoholics Anonymous
Grand Central Station
P.O. Box 459
New York, NY 10163
www.aa.org

Alcoholics Anonymous is a nonsectarian self-help fellowship of men and women working together to recover from alcoholism. There are no dues or fees for membership. Check the group's website for local chapter meetings and information about programs for adults and teens, alcoholism, and the challenges of living with an alcoholic. First-responder-only meeting times and locations in the United States can be found at www.policesuicidestudy.com/id27.html.

Al-Anon Family Group Headquarters
1600 Corporate Landing Parkway
Virginia Beach, VA 23454-5617
Phone: 888-4AL-ANON, Monday–Friday, 8:00 A.M.–6:00 P.M. EST, for meeting information.
www.al-anon.org
e-mail: WSO@al-anon.org

This organization exists to help families and friends of alcoholics cope with the effects of living with the problem drinking of a relative or friend. Alateen is their program for young people. Check the website for information, services, and reading materials

Brattleboro Retreat Uniformed Services Program
www.brattlebororetreat.org

This program in Brattleboro, Vermont, offers inpatient and outpatient treatment for emergency responders struggling with addictions, substance abuse, and PTSD.

Marworth Treatment Center
www.marworth.org

Based in Waverly, Pennsylvania, Marworth offers an inpatient uniformed services program for police officers and fire fighters who need treatment for alcohol and chemical dependency.

National Drug and Alcohol Treatment Referral Routing Service

This service of the U.S. Department of Health and Human Services Substance Abuse and Mental Health Services Administration provides a toll-free telephone number: 1-800-662-HELP.

National Institute on Alcohol Abuse and Alcoholism
5635 Fishers Lane, MSC 9304
Bethesda, MD 20892-9304
www.niaaa.nih.gov/

NIAAA's website has links to other organizations, referral/treatment information, publications, and information about recent research.

www.nlm.nih.gov/medlineplus/alcoholism.html

This is an excellent, easy-to-use online resource for information and referrals.

Narcotics Anonymous (NA World Services)
P.O. Box 9999
Van Nuys, CA 91409
Phone: 818-773-9999
www.na.org

This worldwide, no-cost, self-help organization is akin to Alcoholics Anonymous. It is active in over 100 countries and has about 30,000 meetings in the United States. You can locate a meeting near you or access their help lines by visiting their website.

Publications

Black, C. (1982). *It will never happen to me.* Denver: MAC.

A classic book for adult children of alcoholics.

Liptak, J., & Leutenberg, E. (2008). *Substance abuse and recovery workbook.* Duluth, MN: Whole Person Associates.
A workbook for those struggling with abuse and co-dependence.

Tips for first responders: Possible alcohol and substance abuse indicators. SAMHSA.
A free brochure with a list of indicators associated with substance abuse and physical and mental concerns. Lists a number of signs that may suggest a referral is needed. Pub id: NMH05-0212. Available from www.store.samhsa.gov.

DIVERSITY

Organizations

International Association of Fire Chiefs—Human Relations Committee
4025 Fair Ridge Drive, Suite 300
Fairfax, VA 22033-2868
Phone: 703-273-0911
www.iafc.org

The mission of the Human Relations Committee is to identify human relations and diversity issues and develop and promote solutions to assist the fire serve in achieving a diverse workforce.

International Association of Fire Fighters—Human Relations Committee
1750 New York Avenue NW
Washington, DC 20006
Phone: 202-737-8484
www.iaff.org

The Human Relations Committee was established in 1987. The IAFF holds conferences and has a human relations manual that can be downloaded from its website.

International Association of Women in Fire & Emergency Services
  (iWomen)
4025 Fair Ridge Drive, Suite 300
Fairfax, VA 22033
Phone: 703-896-4858, 4025
e-mail: staff@i-women.org

This organization resulted from a merger of the Women in the Fire Service and Women Chief Fire Officers. Its mission is to provide a proactive network that supports, mentors, educates, and advocates for current and future women in the fire and emergency services. It sponsors conferences, and its website is crammed with intelligent, well written, informative articles and a rich list of links of interest to women in the emergency response professions.

National Association of Hispanic Firefighters
725 Timberhill Drive
Hurst, TX 76053
Phone: 817-905-3312

This organization represents approximately 20,000 paid and volunteer Hispanic fire fighters. It offers support, education, training, and networking with the goal of promoting the recruitment, retention, and advancement of Hispanic fire fighters. It also works to promote fire safety within Hispanic communities.

International Association of Black Professional Fire Fighters
1200 G Street NW
Suite 800
Washington, DC 20005
Phone: 877-213-2170
Fax: 202-434-8707
www.iabpff.org

Founded in 1969, this organization has 5,000 members. It's purpose is to create a global network among black fire fighters, to assist in their recruitment and advancement, to collect and evaluate data on deleterious conditions in areas where minorities live, to compile information concerning the social injustices that exist in the application of working conditions in the fire service, and to implement action to correct them.

FireFLAG/EMS
208 West 13th Street
New York, NY 10011
Phone: 917-885-0127
www.fireflag.org

FireFLAG/EMS is a national peer support group for gay and bisexual
fire fighters, EMTs, and paramedics.

Fire Brigades Union Gay and Lesbian Support Group
Bradley House
68 Coombe Road
Kingston-upon-Thames
Surrey KT2 7AE, UK
Phone: 0208 541 1765
www.fbulgbt.org.uk

This group was established by gay and lesbian fire fighters who are
"out" at work and in a position to help others within the U.K. fire service. They offer confidential support and advice to those who feel isolated or harassed.

Parents, Families and Friends of Lesbians and Gays (PFLAG)
1828 L Street NW, Suite 660
Washington, DC 20036
Phone: 202-467-8180
Fax: 202-467-8194
www.pflag.org

PFLAG is a grassroots organization of more than 55,000 families that
offers support, education, and advocacy. It publishes a newspaper and
holds annual conferences.

Websites

www.facebook.com/FemaleFirefightersSisterhood

A Facebook page offering support and information for female fire fighters with news, relevant articles, and personal stories.

www.fitting-in.com

This British website is managed by retired fire fighter Dr. Dave Baigent and dedicated to publishing research on the fire service. There are a variety of articles and scholarly papers on technical and cultural topics. Of particular interest are Dr. Baigent's study, "The Social Construction of Masculinity in the Fire Service" (2001), and L. Wood's unpublished master's thesis (2002), "A Sociological Exploration of the Occupational Culture of the Fire Service and Women's Place within It."

www.nwfs.net

The website of the British women fire fighters' organization known as Networking Women in the Fire Service.

Books and Reports

Berkman, B., Floren, T., & Willing, L. (1999, November). *Many women strong: A handbook for women fire fighters* (USFA EME-5-4651). Available from Women in the Fire Service, P.O. Box 5446, Madison, WI 53705; phone: 608-233-4768 or order online: www.wfsi.org.

This is a "must read" for current and prospective women fire fighters, whether in the career, volunteer, or wildland service. It is packed with information and resources pertinent to women's health and success in the fire service.

Chetkovich, C. (1997). *Real heat: Gender and race in the urban fire service*. Piscataway, NJ: Rutgers University Press.

This book is an adaptation of Dr. Chetkovich's dissertation; as such it is a challenging, but important, read for any minority male or female in the fire service or thinking of joining the fire service. It also should be mandatory for fire service managers and diversity trainers.

Hagen, S., & Carouba, M. (2002). *Women at Ground Zero: Stories of courage and compassion*. Indianapolis: Alpha Books.

This truly beautiful book written by a fire fighter and social worker is filled with photos and stories from women fire fighters, police officers, medics, and EMTs who responded to the World Trade Center on 9/11. Women's experiences were all but ignored by the media, who focused exclusively on "firemen" and "policemen" despite the fact that three women—an EMT and two police officers—died at the scene.

Health and Safety Issues of the Female Emergency Responder. (1994). FEMA, USFA.

This report is based on issues stemming from a 1994 conference on this topic. Available online: www.usfa.dhs.gov/downloads/pdf/publications/fa-162.pdf.

Hulett, D., Bendick, M., Thomas, S., & Moccio F. (2008). *A national report card on women in firefighting.* Available from Google Books.

This research project was carried out by the Employment Justice Research Center in conjunction with Cornell University and the Ford Foundation. The project documented the experiences of women fire fighters nationwide.

U.S. Department of Homeland Security & FEMA. (4/24/2013). *Many women strong: A handbook for women firefighters.*

This handbook was created to help women who would like to become career, volunteer, or seasonal fire fighters, as well as those who have just started on the job and are seeking guidance. It offers insights and suggestions from women who have been there: female fire fighters, officers, and chiefs from all across the country. This and other similar reports may be downloaded for free at www.i-women.org/reports.php.

Videos

Test of courage: The making of a fire fighter. (2000).

A one-hour documentary about men and women from diverse backgrounds striving to become fire fighters. Filmed in 2000 in Oakland, California, the story shows how these aspiring fire fighters navigate cultural divides to learn to live and work together while meeting the daily pressures of saving lives. Available from The Working Group, www.theworkinggroup.org; Phone: 510-268-9675; e-mail: info@theworkinggroup.org. It costs $99.

Some Real Heat (director/producer: S. Jordan@snafu.de). (2001).

A hard-hitting documentary about six female fire fighters in San Francisco. The women speak candidly about their experiences and the myths and realities of their chosen profession. Available from Women Make Movies, 115 W. 29th Street, Suite 1200, New York, NY 10001; phone: 212-925-0606; e-mail: orders@wmm.com; or order online: www.wmm.com.

A tale of "O": On being different.

This is an animated video that looks at the experience of being one of the few—an "O" among "X's." It explores the consequences of being different without finger pointing—everyone can identify. A discussion guide and a leader's manual are also available. Available from TrainingABC; Phone: 888-281-8038; www.trainingabc.com.

Conferences and Consultants

Linda F. Willing
P.O. Box 148
Grand Lake, CO 80447
Phone: 970-627-3732
e-mail: linda@rwtraining.com
website: www.rwtraining.com

Linda Willing was a career fire fighter and fire officer for over 18 years. Her organization, RealWorld Training & Consulting, offers consultation and training for fire and emergency services that are seeking assistance with conflict resolution and mediation, recruitment and retention, building diverse teams, harassment and discrimination prevention. Her website contains a lot of practical and useful information and reading.

The Carl Holmes Executive Development Institute
https://edionline.net

This five-year (300-hour) executive development program was founded by retired Oklahoma City fire chief Dr. Carl Holmes to promote training and opportunity for minority fire fighters seeking career advancement and personal development. Students meet onsite one week per year at Dillard University in New Orleans, Louisiana.

DOMESTIC VIOLENCE

National Domestic Violence Hotline: 1-800-799-SAFE

Go to the organization's secure website, www.thehotline.org, for information, including advice about safety plans and links to other organizations and online resources.

FAMILY MATTERS

Organizations

International Association of Fire Chiefs
4025 Fair Ridge Drive, Suite 300
Fairfax, VA 22033-2868
Phone: 703-273-0911
www.iafc.org

The International Association of Fire Chiefs usually has a "Partner's Program" and hospitality suite at their annual conference. Activities and topics vary from year to year but are designed to be of interest to spouses and families.

Gottman Institute
1401 East Jefferson Street, Suite 501
Seattle, WA 98122
Phone: 888-523-9042
www.gottman.com

The Gottman Institute is renowned for high-quality, research-based marital therapy. Visit its website, where you can take a relationship quiz, read self-help tips, get information about couples weekend workshops, and referrals to Gottman-trained therapists throughout the United States.

Websites

http://firefighterwife.com

This site provides helpful resources to strengthen the fire family, a network of fire wife blogs, a private chat group, monthly topics such as fitness, marriage builders, home improvement, parenting, finances, book clubs, etc., and local meet-ups so you can connect in person with fire wives in your area.

www.wildlandfirefighterwives.blogspot.com

The motto for this website and blog is "If you think it's tough being a wildland fire fighter . . . try being a wildland fire fighter's wife!"

The Ready Responder
www.ready.gov

The Federal Emergency Management Agency offers a number of comprehensive, free online toolkits to help first responders and their families prepare for emergencies. For example, the Ready Responder toolkit includes a family communication plan to fill out at home, ideas about assisting family members with special needs, information on how to shut off utilities, and help with planning for emergencies at school or work.

usfa.fema.gov

Includes information about disaster planning and keeping your family safe from fire and natural disasters.

Books and Publishers

Farren, S. (2005). *The fireman's wife: A memoir.* New York: Hyperion.

Gottman, J. (1994). *Why marriages succeed or fail and how you can make yours last.* New York: Simon & Schuster.
Gottman, J. (1999). *The seven principles for making marriage work.* New York: Crown.
Gottman, J., & Silver, N. (2013). *What makes love last? How to build trust and avoid betrayal.* New York: Simon & Schuster.

I like John Gottman's many books. They are practical, readable, and based on good research from his "love lab." Some come with exercises and self assessment questionnaires. Try these three for a start.

Lerner, H. (1985). *The dance of anger.* New York: Harper & Row.
Lerner, H. (1989). *The dance of intimacy.* New York: Harper & Row.

Lerner has written many self-help and relationship books, but these two classics are among my favorites. They are written for women, but I think they also apply to men. They are compassionate and filled with practical wisdom and understanding.

Sussman, J., & Glakas-Tenet, S. (2002). *Dare to repair: A do it herself guide to fixing (almost) anything in the home.* New York: HarperResource.

An illustrated guide written by two women whose husbands' public safety jobs kept them away from home.

Magination Press
750 First Street NE
Washington, DC 20002-4242
Phone: 800-374-2721
www.maginationpress.com

Magination Press, a division of the American Psychological Association, publishes books for children and teens that tackle tough issues like loneliness, grief, anxiety, trauma, divorce, and difficult emotions.

New Harbinger Press
5674 Shattuck Avenue
Oakland, CA 94609
Phone: 800-748-6273 or 510-652-0215
Fax: 510-652-5472
www.newharbinger.com

This publishing house specializes in quality self-help books for the public. Consult their website for a list of their publications.

HEALTH AND SAFETY

Organizations

National Fire Protection Association (NFPA)
1 Batterymarch Park
Quincy, MA 02169-7471
Phone: 617-770-3000
www.nfpa.org

This international nonprofit organization advocates fire prevention and public safety. It is a valuable source of data collection and information on fire fighter safety. Its fact-filled website has information for fire service professionals and the public.

International Register of Firefighters with Diabetes
www.irfduk.net

Originally intended for operational fire service employees, the IRFD, located in London, has expanded to challenge any unfair employment practices that are imposed upon people with diabetes.

Amputee Firefighters Association
David Dunville, Director
1903 Phoenix Court
Hartland, MI 48453
Phone: 248-889-4311
e-mail: ampfireassoc@aol.com
http://amputeefirefightersassociation.webs.com

This organization's mission is to mentor, support, and assist public safety employees who have lost a limb or face the prospect of losing a limb, with the goal of helping many to return to work.

Redmond Foundation
1750 New York Avenue NW, 3rd floor
Washington, DC 20006

The Redmond Foundation is a nonprofit organization established by the IAFF. Its mission is to encourage, fund, and carry on research and education regarding the occupational hazards and diseases associated with fire fighting. It holds multidisciplinary biennial conferences to bring fire service professionals together with experts from occupational medicine, research, and other related fields.

Congressional Fire Services Institute, Fire Services Caucus
900 Second Street NE, Suite 303
Washington, DC 20002
Phone: 202-371-1277
Fax: 202-682-FIRE (3473)
e-mail: update@cfsi.org

Write to your congressperson. The caucus's mission is to educate members of Congress about issues of fire and life safety.

Websites

www.presidentschallenge.org

The President's Challenge Program encourages children and adults to make physical activity a part of daily life. You can call toll-free 800-258-8146, Monday–Friday, 8:00 A.M.–5:00 P.M. EST.

www.MayoClinic.com

This site is my personal favorite for easy-to-search, easy-to-read information and tools on every imaginable health-related subject.

www.eatright.org

This is the website of the American Dietetic Association. Features information and tips about healthy eating, exercise, weight loss, nutrition, and so on.

www.charmeck.org/city/charlotte/fire

The Charlotte, North Carolina, Fire Department's website includes a detailed explanation, instructions, and photos of the entire candidate physical agility test. Go to the address above, then click on Employment Opportunities and CPAT.

http://safetyandhealthyweek.org

The International Association of Fire Chiefs and the National Volunteer Firefighters Council have partnered to promote the health and safety of all fire fighters. This jam-packed website has excellent resources in a range of topics including physical and behavioral health, suicide prevention, and much more.

Wildland Firefighting

www.fs.fed.us/fire/safety/index.html
www.wffoundation.org
www.iawfonline.org

For information on wildland fire-fighting safety, check out the websites, respectively, of the U.S. Forest Service, the Federal Emergency Management Agency, the Wildland Firefighter Foundation, and the International Association of Wildland Fire (which also publishes *Wildfire* magazine).

LINE-OF-DUTY DEATHS

The National Fallen Firefighters Foundation
P.O. Drawer 498
Emmitsburg, MD 21727
Phone: 301-447-1365
www.firehero.org

The National Fallen Firefighters Foundations sponsors the annual National Fallen Firefighters Memorial Weekend and Memorial Walk of Honor at the National Fallen Firefighters Memorial in Emmitsburg, Maryland. The foundation provides information, booklets, brochures, and person-to-person support for departments and families coping with a line-of-duty death (LODD). It sponsors a six-hour training program titled "Taking Care of Our Own" that helps senior officers prepare their departments for a LODD. Check its website for a complete description of services, which range from practical advice for conducting funerals to emotional guidance for the bereaved. (See Chapter 8 for more information on the NFFF.)

National Institute for Occupational Safety and Health (NIOSH)
1600 Clifton Road
Atlanta, GA 30333
Phone: 1-800-232-4636
www.cdc.gov/niosh/fire

This website has information on fire fighter fatalities including incident reports, investigations, prevention programs, tips regarding health and safety, and links to other fire-related sites.

www.firehouse.com

This huge website is filled with information of all kinds. It features every fire fighter line-of-duty death (LODD) in the United States and elsewhere, along with civilian fire deaths. If you are so inclined, they will send you an e-mail alert for every LODD.

Compassionate Friends
P.O. Box 3696
Oak Brook, IL 60522-3696
Phone: 630-990-0010; toll free: 877-969-0010
www.compassionatefriends.org

Compassionate Friends is a national, nonprofit, self-help, support organization that offers friendship, understanding, and hope to bereaved parents, grandparents, and siblings. It is nonsectarian and requires no membership dues or fees. Go to the group's website for support, referral, and information on bereavement.

Everyone Goes Home

Everyone Goes Home is a program by the National Fallen Firefighters Foundation to prevent fire fighter line-of-duty deaths and injuries. In March 2004 a Firefighter Life Safety Summit was held to address the need for change within the fire service. At this summit, the 16 Firefighter Life Safety Initiatives were created. Initiative 13, Behavioral Health, offers an array of resources to combat stress, depression, suicide, and PTSD, plus a web-based training course, "Helping Heroes," for providers working with fire fighters.

Books

Carestio, M. (2010). *Black Jack Jetty: A boy's journey through grief.* Washington, DC: Magination Press.

This book follows a young boy as he copes with his father's death and journeys through his grief, anger, anxiety, and guilt.

Kaplow, J., & Pincus, D. (2007). *Samantha Jane's missing smile: A story about coping with the loss of a parent.* Washington, DC: Magination Press.

This book gently guides families through the feelings, thoughts, and wishes that children experience when a parent dies, and offers helpful tools for lasting hope and happiness.

MENTAL HEALTH AND PSYCHOLOGICAL SUPPORT

Organizations

The **National Center for Telehealth and Technology**
www.T2health.org

This organization offers free mobile apps for veterans that are also relevant to first responders who struggle with PTSD or stress management issues. The apps include BioZen (live biofeedback data that requires compatible biosensor devices); Breathe 2 Relax (a portable stress management tool); PTSD Coach (an educational tool for individuals experiencing PTSD symptoms); T2 Mood Tracker (which allows users to self-monitor, track, and reference their emotional experience over time); and Tactical Breather (a tool to help users gain control over physiological and psychological responses to stress).

National Stepfamily Resource Center
www.stepfamilies.info

A national self-help organization with local support groups, educational conferences, and a catalog of books, tapes, and resources for step-families.

National Center for PTSD
www.ptsd.va.gov

This program of the U.S. Department of Veterans Affairs maintains a website that is an educational resource concerning PTSD and other enduring consequences of traumatic stress.

www.cdc.gov/niosh/topics/traumaticincident

The Centers for Disease Control and Prevention and the National Institute for Occupational Safety and Health maintain a page on their website for emergency services responders to learn about traumatic stress. The page has a list of symptoms, links to other sites, and advice on coping at work and at home.

National Mental Health Consumers' Self-Help Clearinghouse
1211 Chestnut Street, Suite 1207
Philadelphia, PA 19107
Phone: 800-553-4539
Fax: 215-636-6312
e-mail: info@mhselfhelp.org
www.mhselfhelp.org

As the word "clearinghouse" suggests, this is a resource for information and referral to mental health self-help groups and organizations.

Project Resilience
5410 Connecticut Avenue NW, Suite 113
Washington, DC 20015
www.projectresilience.com

Project Resilience is a private organization that promotes resilience and resilience training. It maintains an easy-to-navigate website about resilience with many resources.

American Psychological Association Help Center
750 First Street NE
Washington, DC 20002-4242
Phone: 800-374-2721
www.apa.org/helpcenter

The American Psychological Association sponsors a public website on which you will find guidance and information on many topics relating to psychological health and well-being for adults and children, as well as referral sources and a free brochure titled *The Road to Resilience*. Also on the website is an online version of the Posttraumatic Growth Inventory developed by psychologists Richard Tedeschi and Lawrence Calhoun. This 21-item inventory may help you recognize how you have grown after a challenging time or event and identify sources of strength that you can call on in future challenges. It can also aid you in identifying areas you may want to explore further.

American Psychological Association Disaster Response Network
750 First Street NE
Washington, DC 20002-4242
Phone: 800-374-2721
www.apa.org/practice/programs/drn.index.aspx

This is a nationwide collaborative effort between volunteers from the American Psychological Association and the American Red Cross to provide free onsite mental health services for disaster victims and responding emergency personnel.

Gift from Within
16 Cobb Hill Road
Camden, ME 04843
Phone: 207-236-8858
www.giftfromwithin.org
e-mail: JoyceB3955@aol.com

This private nonprofit organization is dedicated to those who suffer from posttraumatic stress disorder (PTSD), those at risk for PTSD, and those who care for traumatized individuals. It develops and disseminates educational material, including videotapes, articles, books, and other resources, through its website and maintains a roster of survivors who are willing to participate in an international network of peer support.

Book

Greene, P., Kane, D., Christ, G. H., Lynch, S., & Corrigan, M. P. (2006). *FDNY crisis counseling: Innovative responses to 9/11 firefighters, families, and communities.* Hoboken, NJ: Wiley.

REFERRAL AND TREATMENT

Organizations

Atlantic OccuPsych
29 W. Susquehanna Ave.
Suite 704
Towson, MD 21204
Phone: 410-823-0555 or 800-962-5763
e-mail: Curran@AtlanticOccupsych.com

Atlantic OccuPsych provides pre-employment psychological assessment services across the United States. There are more than 150 psychologists, clinical social workers, and other licensed mental health professionals who are ready to respond when traumatic incidents occur in its network.

On Site Academy
P. O. Box 1031
Gardner, MA 01440
Phone: 978-874-0177
www.onsiteacademy.org

This nonprofit, five-day residential program is designed for fire fighters and other emergency responders who have been profoundly affected by traumatic stress. Spouses may be included. The program is facilitated by peers and mental health professionals. Fees include room and board and may be covered by your insurance.

West Coast Post-Trauma Retreat
4460-16 Redwood Highway, #362
San Rafael, CA 94903
Phone: 415-721-9789
www.WCPR2001.org
e-mail: wcpr2001@gmail.com

These confidential five-day residential programs for small groups of emergency responders are staffed by peers, mental health professionals, and chaplains. Residents receive individual and group counseling, educational information, and practical tools for dealing with stress, depression, anxiety, and/or PTSD. The fee includes room and board and may be covered by insurance or worker's compensation benefits. They also offer a two-day program of support, education, and assistance to the spouses/significant others of emergency responders who are coping with stress and critical incidents. This program is staffed by clinicians and spousal peers.

Fire/Police Referral Network
Phone: 888-668-2677
http://cfbnetwork.com/

This is a no-cost, nationwide referral program. Participating providers have been screened to ensure documented professional commitment and experience counseling fire fighters and their families.

International Critical Incident Stress Foundation
3290 Pine Orchard Lane, Suite 106
Ellicott City, MD 21042
Phone: 410-750-9600; emergency phone: 410-313-2473
www.icisf.org
e-mail: info@icisf.org

The International Critical Incident Stress Foundation (ICISF) is dedicated to the prevention and mitigation of disabling stress for all emergency services professions through the provision of education, training, support services, and consultation in the establishment of crisis and disaster response programs. Visit its website for a calendar of training conferences, classes, and publications.

Safe Call Now
www.Safecallnow.org

This nonprofit corporation provides crisis intervention and referral services to public safety employees and their families. The 24-hour confidential hotline at 206-459-3020 is staffed by public safety professionals and culturally competent mental health providers.

STRESS MANAGEMENT

Books

Hopson, J., Hopson, E., & Dyar, J. (2001). *Burnout to balance: EMS stress*. Englewood Cliffs, NJ: Prentice-Hall.

Excellent book loaded with practical tips for coping with job stress and building support for yourself at work and at home. Special instructions for EMS workers, family members, supervisors, and instructors.

Goleman, D. (2005). *Emotional intelligence*. New York: Bantam Books.

Goleman, D. (2000). *Working with emotional intelligence*. New York: Bantam Books.

These two readable books demonstrate why emotional know-how matters more than IQ at home and at work.

Greenberger, D., & Padesky, C. (1995). *Mind over mood*. New York: Guilford Press.

This write-in workbook is easy to read and understand. Solidly grounded in research, it will help you identify and then change the thoughts that contribute to your problems.

Davis, M., McKay, M., & Eshelman, E. (2008). *The relaxation and stress reduction handbook*. Oakland, CA: New Harbinger.

A comprehensive stress management workbook now in its fifth edition. It includes ideas for mastering self-care strategies such as time management, assertiveness, meditation, nutrition, and exercise.

Dietz, T. (2009). *Scenes of compassion: A responder's guide for dealing with emergency scene emotional crisis*. Maryland: Chevron Publishing.

The author is an experienced medic and counselor who rightly believes that learning how to deal with victims makes the responders' job easier and reduces stress and compassion fatigue.

Matsakis, A. (1992). *I can't get over it: A handbook for trauma survivors*. Oakland, CA: New Harbinger.

A handbook for people with PTSD, their families, and their friends. It helps survivors cope with memories and emotions, explains secondary wounding, and identifies the triggers that reactivate traumatic stress. It contains lots of practical ideas and advice for recovery and an excellent resource section.

Matsakis, A. (2005). *In harm's way: Help for the wives of military men, police, EMTs, & firefighters*. Oakland, CA: New Harbinger.

Matsakis, A. (2014). *Loving someone with PTSD: A practical guide to understanding and connecting with your partner after trauma*. Oakland, CA: New Harbinger.

U.S. Department of Health and Human Services. *Managing stress: A guide for emergency response workers.*

A free brochure with stress-prevention and management tips for first responders. Available from store.samhsa.gov, publication number NMH05-0211.

SUICIDE

Organizations

American Foundation for Suicide Prevention
120 Wall Street, 29th Floor
New York, NY 10005
Toll-free phone: 888-333-AFSP
Phone: 212-363-3500
website: www.afsp.org
e-mail: inquiry@afsp.org

This advocacy group seeks to promote research and raise public awareness about suicide. Their informative website includes information and referral resources for survivors of suicide.

National Hopeline Network
Phone: 1-800-SUICIDE, 1-800-784-2433
www.hopeline.com

This toll-free hotline works 24/7. The website has online crisis support, information, and referral resources.

VOLUNTEERS

Organization

National Volunteer Fire Council
7852 Walker Drive, Suite 375
Greenbelt, MD 20770
202-887-5700; 1-888-ASK-NVFC
www.nvfc.org

The National Volunteer Fire Council (NVFC) is a nonprofit membership association representing the interests of the volunteer fire, EMS, and rescue services. The NVFC serves as an information source regarding legislation, standards, and regulatory issues. Its website features volunteer opportunities, legislative updates, and links to other sites.

Books

Perry, M. (2002). *Population: 485. Meeting your neighbors one siren at a time.* New York: HarperCollins.

A beautifully written memoir about life in a small Wisconsin town as seen through the eyes of a volunteer fire fighter.

Fire Chaplains

Federation of Fire Chaplains
PO Box 437
Meridian, TX 76665
Phone: 254-435-2256
www.firechaplains.org

Their website has information on starting a chaplaincy program in your department.

Bibliography

INTRODUCTION

Beil, K. (1999). *Fire in their eyes: Wildfires and the people who fight them.* New York: Harcourt Brace.

Casstevens, D. (2000, May 5). Brunacini taking good care of "Mrs. Smith." *The Arizona Republic*, p. 19.

Chard, P. S. (1987, January–February). Grief: Handling theirs and yours. *Emergency Medical Services*, 16, 36–38, 40–43.

Dobson, J. (1994). *Seven promises of a promise keeper.* Colorado Springs, CO: Focus of the Family.

Flynn, S. (2002). *3000 degrees: The true story of a deadly fire and the men who fought it.* New York: Warner.

Frazier, S. (1996, August). *A guide for fire officers to improve their skills and abilities as both husbands and fathers.* An applied research project submitted to the National Fire Academy as part of the Executive Fire Officer Program. (Available on interlibrary loan at *www.lrc.fema.gov*)

Gist, R., & Lubin, B. (Eds.). (1989). *Psychosocial aspects of disaster.* New York: Wiley.

Hartsough, D., & Myers, D. (1985). *Disaster work and mental health: Prevention and control of stress among workers.* New York: Brunner/Mazel.

Hokanson, M. (1997, February). *Evaluation of the effectiveness of the CISM Program for the Los Angeles County Fire Department.* An applied research project submitted to the National Fire Academy as part of the Executive Fire Officer Program. (Available on interlibrary loan at *www.lrc.fema.gov*)

271

Miletich, J. J. (1990). *Police, firefighter and paramedic stress: An annotated bibliography.* New York: Greenwood Press.

Mulcare, T. (1998). Why they do what they do: Traits among firefighters and paramedics. *Health and Safety, 9*(10), 13–14.

Pfefferbaum, B., North, C. S., Bunch, K., Wilson, T. G., Tucker, P., & Schorr, J. K. (2002). The impact of the 1995 Oklahoma City bombing on the partners of firefighters. *Journal of Urban Health: Bulletin of the New York Academy of Medicine, 79*(3), 364–372.

Sauter, S., & Murphy, L. (Eds.). (1995). *Organizational risk factors for job stress.* Washington, DC: American Psychological Association.

Scharfenberg, J. (1989, August). *Critical incident stress as it relates to the executive fire officer: An investigative review.* An applied research project submitted to the National Fire Academy as part of the Executive Fire Officer Program. (Available on interlibrary loan at *www.lrc.fema.gov*)

Smith, R. (2002, February 1). How to balance the two families of firefighting. *Fire Chief.* Available at http://firechief.com/issue_20020201

Woodall, S. J. (1993, July). *Emergency worker stress assessment survey development.* An applied research project submitted to the National Fire Academy as part of the Executive Fire Officer Program. (Available on interlibrary loan at *www.lrc.fema.gov*)

CHAPTER 1

Barnett, R. C., & Hyde, J. S. (2001). Women, men, work, and family: An expansionist theory. *American Psychologist, 56*(10), 781–796.

Beaton, R., Murphy, S., Pike, K., & Corneil, W. (1997). Social support and network conflict in firefighters and paramedics. *Western Journal of Nursing Research, 19*(3), 297–313.

Brewer, M., & Weber, J. (1994). Self-evaluation effects of interpersonal versus intergroup social comparison. *ournal of Personality and Social Psychology, 66*(2), 268–275.

Carr, D. (2003, March 23). Rebutting an account of tarnished valor. *New York Times,* p. 31.

Dickenson, C., Dionne, J., Earl, R., Kapler, D., Lewis, K., Tomberg, T., & Westbrook, H. (1985, September). Firefighter! Where is your family when disaster strikes? *American Fire Journal,* pp. 26–46.

Dunn, S. (1991, July). The other side of the story. Emergency Medical Services, 20(7), 27–31.

Figgins, D. L. (1990, May). *Does the 24 hour shift cause divorce in the fire*

272

service? An applied research project for Strategic Analysis of Fire Department Operations at the National Fire Academy. (Available from the author at 716 East Oak St., Bozeman, MT 59715)

Hildebrand, J. (1987, Summer). Job stress and the family: An interview with seven married women. *IAFC Journal*, pp. 26–31.

Langewiesche, W. (2002). *American ground: Unbuilding the World Trade Center.* New York: Point Press.

Marcucci, P. (2001, June). *When dad is a firefighter: Paternal involvement, parental satisfaction and child's well being.* Unpublished doctoral dissertation, Alliant University.

McCallion, R., & Fazackerly, J. (1991, October). Burning the EMS candle: EMS shifts and worker fatigue. *Emergency Medical Services*, 16(10), 40–47.

McDermott, T. (1997, November). *Anxiety in families of fire fighters: Recognition and response.* An applied research project for Strategic Analysis of Fire Department Operations at the National Fire Academy. (Available from the author at 515 North 7th St., Rochelle, IN 61068)

Murphy, S. A., Beaton, R., Cain, K., & Pike, K. (1994). Gender diferences in fire fighter job stressors and symptoms of stress. *Women and Health*, 22(2), 55–69.

Noran, A. R. (1995). Literature search on the wives of firefighters. *Employee Assistance Quarterly*, 10(3), 65–79.

Paley, M. J., & Tepas, D. I. (1994). Fatigue and the shiftworker: Firefighters working on a rotating shift schedule. *Human Factors*, 36(2), 269–284.

Smith, D. (2002, July–August). Making work your family's ally. *American Psychological Association Monitor on Psychology*, 33(7), 58.

CHAPTER 2

Corneil, W. (1991, March). Fire department trauma. *Employee Assistance Magazine*, pp. 28–34.

Flynn, S. (2002). *3000 degrees: The true story of a deadly fire and the men who fought it.* New York: Warner.

Gottman, J. (1994). *Why marriages succeed or fail.* New York: Fireside.

Hibbard, J. (1997). Little red book of firehouse pranks (Vol. 1). (Available from the author at 13237 Sierra Highway, Saugus, CA 91350)

James, S. (2003, May 30). Two Florida firefighters lose jobs over hazing incident. *Sun Sentinal.* Available at www.firehouse.com

Kirschman, E. (1997). *I love a cop: What police families need to know.* New York: Guilford press.

Phillips, S. R. (1996). *Creating effective relationships.* Carlsbad, CA: Personal Strengths Publishing.

Slater, L. (2003, February 23). Repress yourself. *New York Times Magazine,* p. 48.

CHAPTER 3

Elshaug, C., & Metzer, J. (2001). Personality attributes of volunteers and paid workers engaged in similar occupational tasks. *Journal of Social Psychology, 141*(6), 752

Hui, L., Arvey, R. D., & Butler, R. (2001). Correlates of work injury frequency and duration among firefighters. *Journal of Occupational Health Psychology, 6*(3), 229–242.

McIntosh, N. (1995). Exhilarating work: An antidote for dangerous work?" In S. Sauter & L. Murphy (Eds.), *Organizational risk factors for job stress* (pp. 303–316). Washington, DC: American Psychological Association.

Wambaugh, J. (1992). A jury of one. In *From the files of Joseph Wambaugh* [TV series]. New York: National Broadcasting Company.

CHAPTER 4

Ballachey, C. (2002). Unpublished study. (Available from the author at P.O. Box 7515, Berkeley, CA 94707)

Bass, R. (2000, Spring). Fireman. *Kenyon Review,* pp. 11–29.

Benest, F., & Grijalva, R. (2002, January–February). Enhancing the manager/fire chief relationship. *Public Management,* pp. 6–9.

Coleman, R. J. (1998). *Going for gold.* Albany, NY: Delmar.

Coleman, R. J. (1999, August 1). Blinded by the gold's glare: The reality of being chief. *Fire Chief.* Available at www.firechief.com

Gater, L. (1999, October). Red hot jobs in firefighting. *Career World,* pp. 22–26.

Milligan, A. (2004, April). *Calpers experience study, 1997–2002.* Available at www.calpers.ca.gov

Nelson, A. (2002). *The guys: A play.* New York: Random House.

Polgreen, L. (2003, January 16). O.K., chief, it's time to get down to business. *New York Times,* p. 3.

Buckman, J. (2002, September). The future of the volunteer fire service. *Fire Engineering*, p. 10.

Muegge, C., Zollinger, T., Saywell, R., Moffatt, S., Hanify, T., & Deelan, L. (2002, August). CPAT: Putting the test to the test. *Fire Engineering*, pp. 97–102.

Carrell, J., & Moore, T. (1999, May). Training to slay the dragon. *Smithsonian*, pp. 100–110.

Firefighters accused of hazing female coworker won't face charges. (2003, April 22). *Available at www.firehouse.com*

Lewis, W. (2001, February). Developing and implementing a mentor program. *Fire Engineering*, pp. 61–69.

Prentice, D., & Miller, D. (2002, May). The emergence of homegrown stereotypes. *American Psychologist*, pp. 352–359.

Scharfenberg, J. (1989, August). *Critical incident stress as it relates to the executive fire officer: An investigative review.* An applied research project submitted to the National Fire Academy as part of the Executive Fire Officer Program. (Available on interlibrary loan at *www.lrc.fema.gov*)

Schmader, D. (2002, March 11 and April 11). *Last Days: The week in review.* Available at *www.thestranger.com*.

Stoddard, M. G. (2002). The art of the firefighter. *Saturday Evening Post*, 274(2), 54.

CHAPTER 5

Beaton, R. D., & Murphy, S. A. (1995). Working with people in crisis: Research implications. In C. Figley (Ed.), *Compassion fatigue* (pp. 51–81). New York: Brunner-Routledge.

Corneil, W., Beaton, R., Murphy, S., Johnson, C., & Pike, K. (1999). Exposure to traumatic incidents and prevalence of posttraumatic stress symptomatology in urban firefighters in two countries. *Journal of Occupational Health Psychology*, 4(2), 131–141.

Dunn, S. (1991, July). The other side of the story. *Emergency Medical Services*, 20(7), 27–31.

Dutton, L., Smolensky, M., Leach, C., Lorimor, R., & Hsi, B. (1978). Stress levels of ambulance paramedics and fire fighters. *Journal of Occupational Medicine*, 20(2), 111–115.

Fischman, J. (1984, February). Trauma junkies. *Psychology Today*, p. 79.

Genest, M., Levine, J., Ramsden, V., & Swanson, R. (1990). The impact of providing help: Emergency workers and cardiopulmonary resuscitation attempts. *Journal of Traumatic Stress*, 3(2), 305–313.

Heightman, A. (2002, August). From the Editor. *Emergency Medical Services*, p. 10.

Hopson, J., Hopson, E., & Dyar, J. (2001). Burnout to balance: EMS stress. Upper Saddle River, NJ: Prentice Hall.

Marmar, C., Weiss, D., Metzler, M., DeLucchi, K., Best, S., & Wentworth, K. (1999). Longitudinal course and predictors of continuing distress following critical incident exposure in emergency services personnel. *Journal of Nervous and Mental Disease, 187*(1), 15–22.

National Fire Protection Association. (2002, December). *A needs assessment of the U.S. fire service: A cooperative study authorized by U.S. Public Law 106-398* (FA-240). Available at *NFPA.org/research/index/asp.*

Onieal, D. (2002, August). *Diversity in the fire service.* Workshop presented at the Diversity and Equity Conference, Norfolk, VA.

Wallace, M., & Brightmire, S. (1999, September). Fire department response to the Columbine tragedy. *Fire Engineering*, pp. 71–78.

Woodall, J. (1997, January). *Hearts on fire: An ethnographic exploration of the emotional world of firefighters.* Unpublished master's thesis, Ottawa University.

CHAPTER 7

Beaton, R., Johnson, L. C., Infield, S., Ollis, T., & Bond, G. (2001). Outcomes of a leadership intervention for a metropolitan fire department. *Psychological Reports, 88*, 1049–1066.

Beaton, R., & Murphy, S. (1993). Sources of occupational stress among firefighter/EMTs and firefighter/paramedics and correlations with job-related outcomes. *Prehospital and Disaster Medicine, 8*(2), 140–150.

Beaton, R., Murphy, S., Pike, K., & Jarred, M. (1995). Stress symptom factors in firefighters and medics. In S. Sauter & L. Murphy (Eds.), *Organizational risk factors for job stress* (pp. 227–246). Washington, DC: American Psychological Association.

Benoit, J., & Perkins, K. (2000, July). *Managing conflict in combination fire departments* (ICMA Service Report, Vol. 32, No. 7). Available at *www.bookstore.icma.org*

Buckman, J. (1999, August). Responding to a problem firefighter. *Fire Engineering*, pp. 16–18.

Coleman, R. J. (2002, February 1). Have you found a conflict-free combination? *Fire Chief.* Available at *www.firechief.com*

Franklin, B. (1987). Brave men at fires. In J. A. L. LeMay (Ed.), *Benjamin*

276

Franklin: Writings (pp. 220–223). New York: Literary Classics of the United States. (Original work published 1773)

Freedman, A. (1998, September). Camaraderie and organizational dysfunction. *Fire Engineering*, p. 87.

Gist, R., & Woodall, J. (1995). Occupational stress in contemporary fire service. In P. Orris, J. Melius, & R. Duffy (Eds.), *Occupational medicine: Firefighters' safety and health* (Vol. 10, No. 4, pp. 763–787). Philadelphia: Hanley & Belfus.

Litigation: Fire fighters and free speech. (1999, August). *Fire Engineering*, p. 48.

MacAllaster, A. (1989, January). *Stress: It goes beyond the emergency scene.* An applied research project submitted to the National Fire Academy as part of the Executive Fire Officer Program. (Available on interlibrary loan at *www.lrc.fema.gov*)

Martinez, R. J. (1998, April). *The effect of leadership styles on stress indicators in Hawaii's airport firefighting personnel.* An applied research project submitted to the National Fire Academy as part of the Executive Fire Officer Program. (Available on interlibrary loan at *www.lrc.fema.gov*)

National Fire Protection Association, Fire Analysis and Research Division. (2002, December). *Facts about fire: Fire loss in the United States and Canada.* Quincy, MA: Author.

Psychological stress a factor in fire station duty. (2000, December). *Fire Engineering*, p. 28.

Smouldering issues. (1999, November 20). *The Economist*, p. 32f.

Stockwell, J. (2002, February 25). Local firefighters could face choice between 2 passions. *The Washington Post*, p. B1.

CHAPTER 8

Armstrong, D. (1999, February 8). A department under fire. *Boston Globe*.

Armstrong, D., Berkman, B., Floren, T., & Willing, L. (1993, January). *A handbook on women in firefighting: The changing face of the fire service* (USFA FA-128). (Available from WIFS at P.O. Box 5446, Madison, WI 53705 or at www.wfis.org)

Beaton, R. D., Murphy, S. A., Pike, K. C., & Corneil, W. (1997). Social support and network conflict in firefighters and paramedics. *Western Journal of Nursing Research*, 19(3), 297–313.

Berkman, B., Floren, T., & Willing, L. (1999, September). *Many faces, one purpose: A manager's handbook on women in firefighting* (USFA

EME-5-4651). (Available from WIFS at P.O. Box 5446, Madison, WI 53705 or at *www.wfis.org*)

Berkman, B., Floren, T., & Willing, L. (1999, November). *Many women strong: A handbook for women firefighters* (USFA EME-5-4651). (Available from WIFS at P.O. Box 5446, Madison, WI 53705 or at *www.wfis.org*)

Chetkovich, C. (1997). *Real heat: Gender and race in the urban fire service.* New Brunswick, NJ: Rutgers University Press.

Cooper, R. (1995). Fireman: Immaculate manhoood. *Journal of Popular Culture, 28*(4), 139–179.

Floren, T. (1999, September–October). Report on equality in the U.K. fire Service. *Firework* [Newsletter]. Available at *www.wfsi.org*

Her Majesty's Inspectorate of Fire Services. (1999). *Equality and fairness in the fire service: A thematic review.* Available at *www.fbu.org.uk/regions/berkshire/publications/publications.php*

Liao, H., Arvey, R., & Butler, R. (2001, July). Correlates of work injury frequency and duration among firefighters. *Journal of Occupational Health Psychology, 6*(3), 229–242.

Little, J. (2002, June 2). Blacks challenge county fire districts' hiring. *St. Louis Post-Dispatch*, p. A1.

Murphy, S. A., Beaton, R., Cain, K., & Pike, K. (1994). Gender diferences in fire fighter job stressors and symptoms of stress. *Women and Health, 22*(2), 55–69.

One voice speaks for many. (2003, February 1). *Fire Chief* Available at *www.firechief.com*

Partenheimer, D. (2001, July 15). *Two new studies look at role of personality and work demands in health and safety on the job.* APA press release. Available at *www.apa.org/release*

Paul, C. (1998). *Fighting fire.* New York: St. Martin's Press.

Smith, D. (2002, July–August). Making work your family's ally. *American Psychological Association Monitor on Psychology*, p. 58.

Stern, S. (2001, December 3). Women firefighters struggle for first rung. *Christian Science Monitor*, p. 18.

Willing, L. (1996, September). Why we quit. *Firework* [Newsletter]. Available at *www.wfsi.org/arts.quit.html*

Wood, L. (2002). *A sociological exploration of the occupational culture of the fire service and women's place within it.* Master's thesis, University of Edinburgh. Available at www.fittingin.com

WFS survey on women and equipment. (1996, June–August). *Firework* [Newsletter]. Available at *www.wfsi.org*

Yoder, J. D., & Berendsen, L. L. (2001). "Outsider within" the firehouse:

African American and White women firefighters. *Psychology of Women Quarterly*, 25, 27–36.

Health and Safety Issues of the Female Emergency Responder, FEMA/USFA. (1996, June). Available at *www.lrc.fema.gov*

CHAPTER 9

Calvert, G., Merling, J., & Burnett, C. (1999, November). National occupations mortality surveillance system: The association between occupation and ischemic heart disease among 16- to 60-year old males. *Journal of Occupational and Environmental Medicine*, 41(11), 960–966.

Casey, H. (2000, September 28). *Test asks: Can you survive?* Available at *www.firehouse.com*

Choi, B. C. (2000). A technique to reassess epidemiological evidence in light of the healthy worker effect: The case of firefighting and heart disease. *Journal of Occupational and Environmental Medicine*, 42(10), 1021–1034.

Clark, B. A. (2001, October 15). *Mayday, Mayday, Mayday: Do firefighters know when to call it?* Available at *www.firehouse.com*

Clark, B. A. (2002, December). *We have permission to use the word Mayday.* Available at *www.firehouse.com*

Clark, B. A., Auch, S., & Angulo, R. (2002, July). *When would you call Mayday-Mayday-Mayday?* Available at *www.firehouse.com*

Federal Emergency Management Agency. (1998, September). *Aftermath of firefighter fatality incidents: Preparing for the worst.* Available at *www.lrc.fema.gov*

Federal Emergency Management Agency. (2002, April). *Firefighter Fatality Retrospective Study 1990–2000.* Available at *www.lrc.fema.gov*

Firey, C. (2001, March 9). *Oregon firefighters join fitness study.* Available at *www.firehouse.com*

Gertner, J. (2003, September 7). The futile pursuit of happiness. *New York Times Magazine*, p. 44.

Glazner, L. K. (1996). Factors related to injury of shiftworking fire fighters in the Northeastern United States. *Safety Science*, 21, 255–263.

Golden, A., Markowitz, S., & Landrigan, P. (1995). The risk of cancer in firefighters. In P. Orris, J. Melius, & R. Duffy (Eds.), Occupational medicine: Firefighters' safety and health (Vol. 10, No. 4, pp. 803–820). Philadelphia: Hanley & Belfus.

Guidotti, T. L. (1992, February 22). Human factors in firefighting: Ergonomic,cardiopulmonary and psychogenic stress-related issues. *International Archives of Occupational and Environmental Health*, 64(1), 1–12.

Harrison, R., Materna, B., & Rothman, N. (1995). Respiratory health hazards and lung function in wildland firefighters. In P. Orris, J. Melius, & R. Duffy (Eds.), *Occupational medicine: Firefighters' safety and health* (Vol. 10, No. 4, pp. 857–870). Philadelphia: Hanley & Belfus.

Henley, J. (2002, December 2). France weeps for firemen killed by speeding driver. *The Guardian* (London).

International Association of Fire Chiefs. (2002). *Crew resource management: A positive change for the fire service.* Fairfax, VA: Author.

International Association of Fire Chiefs, Health and Safety Committee. (2001, August). *The 10 rules of engagement for structural fire fighting and the acceptability of risk.* Fairfax, VA: Author.

Kales, S. N., Freyman, R., & Hill, J., Polyhronopoulos, G., Aldrich, J., & Christiani, D. (2001). Firefighters' hearing: A comparison with population databases from the International Standards Organization. *Journal of Occupational Environmental Medicine*, 43(7), 650–656.

Kales, S. N., Polyhronopoulos, B., Aldrich, J., Leitao, E., & Christiani, D. (1999). Obesity in Hazmat firefighters. *Journal of Occupational and Environmental Medicine*, 41(6), 589–595.

Kirschman, E. (1997). *I love a cop: What police families need to know.* New York: Guilford Press.

Kirschman, E. (1999, January 28). Adapted from "My Word." *Oakland Tribune.*

Karter, M. J. (2000, February). *Patterns of firefighter fireground injuries.* Quincy, MA: National Fire Protection Association. Available at *www.nfpa.org*

Karter, M. J., & Molis, J. L. (2003). *Firefighter injuries in the United States.* Quincy, MA: National Fire Protection Association. Available at *www.nfpa.org*

LeBlanc, P., & Fahy, R. (2002, July). *Full report: Firefighter fatalities in the United States—2001.* Quincy, MA: National Fire Protection Association. Available at *www.nfpa.org*

Liao, H., Arvey, R., & Butler, R. (2001). Correlates of work injury frequency and duration among firefighters. *Journal of Occupational Health Psychology*, 6(3), 229–242.

McIntosh, N. (1995). Exhilarating work: An antidote for dangerous work?" In S. Sauter & L. Murphy (Eds.), *Organizational risk factors for job stress* (pp. 303–316). Washington, DC: American Psychological Association.

Melius, J. (1995). Cardiovascular disease among firefighters. In P. Orris, J. Melius, & R. Duffy (Eds.), *Occupational medicine: Firefighters' safety and health* (Vol. 10, No. 4, pp. 821–828). Philadelphia: Hanley & Belfus.

Morris, G. (2002, August). *Wellness and risk management.* Presentation at the annual conference of the International Association of Fire Chiefs, Minneapolis, MN.

Murray, D. (2000, February). Study shows firefighters lost their sense of smell. *Safety and Health*, p. 60.

Nagourney, E. (2002, September 10). Patterns: Tandem effects of spouses. *New York Times*, p. 6.

National Fire Protection Association. (2002, December). *A needs assessment of the U.S. fire service: A cooperative study authorized by U.S. Public Law 106-398* (FA-240). Available at *NFPA.org/research/index/asp*

Peabody, Z. (2002, July 1). Column one: Fire polices slide into disuse. *Los Angeles Times*, p. A1.

Pedrola, J. (2001, February). *Managing firefighter death and injury events: Strategic management of change.* An applied research project submitted to the National Fire Academy as part of the Executive Fire Officer Program. (Available from the author at Douglas County Fire District #2, Roseburg, OR 97470)

Peterson, D. F. (2002, August 21). *Firefighting: Risky business: Dealing with the risk of emergency response.* Available at *www.firehouse.com*

Petruzzello, S., & Smith, D. (1996, February). Psychological responses to working in bunker gear. *Fire Engineering*, p. 51.

Phoenix Fire Department. (2002, March 12). *Final report: South West Supermarket fire.* Available at *www.phoenixfire.org*

Reichelt, P., & Conrad, K. (1995). Musculoskeletal injury: Ergonomics and physical fitness in firefighters. In P. Orris, J. Melius, & R. Duffy (Eds.), *Occupational medicine: Firefighters' safety and health* (Vol. 10, No. 4, pp. 735–746). Philadelphia: Hanley & Belfus.

Scannell, C., & Balmes, J. (1995). Pulmonary effects of firefighting. In P. Orris, J. Melius, & R. Duffy (Eds.), *Occupational medicine: Firefighters' safety and health* (Vol. 10, No. 4, pp. 789–802). Philadelphia: Hanley & Belfus.

Schaffer, M. (2001, January 15). Blood, sweat, serious fears. *U.S. New & World Report*, p. 20.

Smith, D., & Petruzello, S. (1998, August). Selected physiological and psychological responses to live fire drills in different gear. *Ergonomics*, *41*(8), 1141.

Smith, D., & Petruzello, S. (2001, February). The effect of strenuous live-fire drills on cardiovascular and psychological responses of recruit firefighters. *Ergonomics, 44*(3), 244.

Stieg, B., & Jones, L. (2002, April). Are you fireman fit? *Men's Health,* p. 50.

Student manual: Rapid intervention crew tactics (2nd ed.). (Available from the California Department of Forestry and Protection, State Fire Training, P.O. Box 944246, Sacramento, CA 94244)

Tubbs. R. (1995). Noise and hearing loss in firefighting. In P. Orris, J. Melius, & R. Duffy (Eds.), *Occupational medicine: Firefighters' safety and health* (Vol. 10, No. 4, pp. 843–856). Philadelphia: Hanley & Belfus.

Upfal, M., Naylor, P., & Mutchnick, M. (2001, April). Anti-hepatitis C virus. *Journal of Occupational and Environmental Medicine, 43*(3), 402–411.

U.S. Centers for Disease Control and Prevention. (2000, July 28). Hepatitis C virus infection among firefighters, emergency medical technicians and paramedics—Selected locations, United States, 1991–2000. *Morbidity and Mortality Weekly Report, 49*(29), 660.

Weaver, V., & Arndt, S. (1995). Communicable disease and firefighters. In P. Orris, J. Melius, & R. Duffy (Eds.), *Occupational medicine: Firefighters' safety and health* (Vol. 10, No. 4, pp. 747–762). Philadelphia: Hanley & Belfus.

Womack, W. (2001, July). Cardiovascular risk markers in firefighters. *Fire Engineering,* p. 24.

CHAPTER 10

American Psychiatric Association. (1994). *Diagnostic and statistical manual of mental disorders* (4th ed., text rev.). Washington, DC: Author.

Baker, S., & Williams, K. (2001). Short communication: Relation between social problem-solving appraisals, work stress and pschological distress in male firefighters. *Stress and Health, 17,* 219–229.

Beaton, R., Murphy, S., Pike, K., & Jarrett, M. (1995). Stress symptom factors in firefighters and paramedics. In S. Sauter & L. Murphy (Eds.), *Organizational risk factors for job stress* (pp. 227–246). Washington, DC: American Psychological Association.

Bonnano, G. (2004, January). Loss, trauma and human resilience: Have we underestimated the human capacity to thrive after extremely aversive events? *American Psychologist,* pp. 20–28.

Calhoun, L., & Tedeschi, R. (2000). Early posttraumatic interventions: Facilitating possibilities for growth. In J. Violanti, D. Paton, & C.

Dunning (Eds.), *Posttraumatic stress intervention: Challenges, issues, and perspectives* (pp. 135–151). Springfield, IL: Charles C. Thomas.

Carlisle, C. (1999, September). *The role of occupational stress in the contemporary fire service: Psychological stress, its causation, identification, treatment, reduction and resolution.* An applied research project submitted to the National Fire Academy as part of the Executive Fire Officer Program. (Available on interlibrary loan at *www.lrc.fema.gov*)

Corneil, W., Beaton, R., Murphy, S., Johnson, C., & Pike, K. (1999). Exposure to traumatic incidents and prevalence of posttraumatic stress symptomatology in urban firefighters in two countries. *Journal of Occupational Health Psychology, 4*(2), 131–141.

Cropper, C. (2002, March 18). When the nightmares won't go away. *Business Week*, p. 106.

Durkin, J., & Bekerian, D. (2000). *Psychological resilience to stress in firefighters.* Unpublished manuscript. Available at www.firestress.co.uk

Figley, C. (Ed.). (1995). *Compassion fatigue.* New York: Brunner/Mazel.

Gist, R. (2002). What have they done to my song?: Social science, social movements and the debriefing debates. *Australasian Journal of Disaster and Trauma Studies* [Online]. Available at *www.massey.ac.nz/trauma*

Gist, R., & Woodall, S. J. (1995). Occupational stress in the contemporary fire service. In P. Orris, J. Melius, & R. Duffy (Eds.), *Occupational medicine: Firefighters' safety and health* (Vol. 10, No. 4, pp. 763–787). Philadelphia: Hanley & Belfus.

Gist, R., & Woodall, S. J. (1998). Social science versus social movements: The origins and natural history of debriefing. *Australasian Journal of Disaster and Trauma Studies* 5[Online]. (Available at *www.massey.ac.nz/trauma*)

Groopman, J. (2004, January 26). The grief industry: How much does crisis counselling help—or hurt? *The New Yorker.* Available at *www.newyorker.com/fact/content*

Guidotti, T. L. (1992, February 22). Human factors in firefighting: Ergonomic, cardiopulmonary and psychogenic stress-related issues. *International Archives of Occupational and Environmental Health, 64*(1), 1–12.

Hemingway, E. (1929). *A farewell to arms.* London: Cape.

Hytten, K., & Hasle, A. (1989). Fire fighters: A study of stress and coping. *Acta Psychiatrica Scandinavica, 355*(Suppl.), 50–55.

Killeen, A. M. (2000, Spring). *Occupatinal stress and coping within the fire department*. Unpublished honors thesis, University of California, Los Angeles.

Larkin, M. (1999, September 18). Can post-traumatic stress disorder be put on hold? *The Lancet, 354,* 1008.

Lifton, J. R., & Olson, E. (1986). The human meaning of total disaster: The Buffalo Creek experience. In R. Moos & J. H. Schaefer (Eds.), *Coping with life crises* (pp. 307–322). New York: Plenum Press.

Marmar, C., Weiss, D., Metzler, M., DeLucchi, K., Best, S., & Wentworth, K. (1999). Longitudinal course and predictors of continuing distress following critical incident exposure in emergency services personnel. *Journal of Nervous and Mental Disease, 187*(1), 15–22.

McClusky, F. (2002). *Thoughts on fire: Life lessons of a volunteer fire-fighter.* Lincoln, NE: Writers Advantage.

McDermott, T. (1997, July). *The fire service response to survivor stress.* An applied research project submitted to the National Fire Academy as part of the Executive Fire Officer Program. (Available on interlibrary loan at *www.lrc.fema.gov*)

McFarlane, A. C. (1988). The phenomenology of posttraumatic stress disorders following a natural disaster. *Journal of Nervous and Mental Disease, 176*(1), 22–29.

McFarlane, A. C. (1992). Aovidance and intrustion in posttraumatic stress disorder. *Journal of Nervous and Mental Disease, 180*(7), 439–445.

McFarlane, A. C. (1998). The aetiology of posttraumatic stress disorders following a natural disaster. *British Journal of Psychiatry, 152,* 116–121.

Murphy, S. A., Bond, G., Beaton, R., Murphy, J., & Johnson, L. C. (2002). Lifestyle practices and occupational stressors as predictors of health outcomes in urban fire fighters. *International Journal of Stress Management, 9*(4), 311–327.

Neylan, T. C., Metzler, T. J., Best, S. R., Weiss, D. S., Fagan, J. A., Liberman, A., Rogers, C., Vedantham, K., Brunet, A., Lipsey, T. L., & Marmar, C. R. (2002). Critical incident exposure and sleep quality in police officers. *Psychosomatic Medicine, 64,* 345–352.

Nixon, S. J., Schorr, J., Boudreaux, A., & Vincent, R. (1999). Perceived sources of support and their effectiveness for Oklahoma City fire-fighters. *Psychiatric Annals, 29*(2), 101–105.

Olson, G. (2003). *The brain and stress.* Unpublished paper. (Available from the author 550 Hamilton Ave., Palo Alto, CA 94301)

Psychological stress a factor in fire station duty. (2000, December). *Fire Engineering,* p. 28.

Regehr, C., Hill, J., & Glancy, G. (2000). Individual predictors of traumatic reactions in firefighters. *Journal of Nervous and Mental Disease*, *188*(6), 333–339.

Tartt, D. (1992). *The secret history.* New York: Ballantine Books.

Violanti, J., Paton, D., & Dunning, C. (Eds.). (2000). *Posttraumatic stress intervention: Challenges, issues, and perspectives.* Springfield, IL: Charles C. Thomas.

Wagner, D., Heinrichs, M., & Ehlert, U. (1998). Prevalence of symptoms of posttraumatic stress disorder in German professional firefighters. *American Journal of Psychiatry, 155,* 1727–1732.

Walsh, F. (1998). *Strengthening family resilience.* New York: Guilford Press.

Woodall, S. J. (1998). *Ask not why the wounded fall, but how the valiant continue to march: New theory on work-related stress management in the fire service.* UMI Dissertation Services. Available at *www. umi.com*

Woodall, S. J. (1997, January). *Hearts on fire: An ethnographic exploration of the emotional world of firefighters.* Unpublished master's thesis, Ottawa University.

CHAPTER 11

Best, S. (2001, October). *The debriefing debate: Research findings and failings.* Presentation at the annual meeting of the International Association of Chiefs of Police, Toronto.

Carlier, I., & Gersons, B. (2000). Brief prevention programs after trauma. In J. Violanti, D. Paton, & C. Dunning (Eds.), *Posttraumatic stress intervention: Challenges, issues, and perspectives* (pp. 65–75). Springfield, IL: Charles C. Thomas.

Disaster mental health: A focus on the long-term. (2001, August 26). Hazards conference, summary of Session #26. Available at *hazctr@spot. colorado.edu*

Emmerik, A. P., Kamphuis, J., Hulsbosch, A., & Emmelkamp, P. (2002, September). Single session debriefing after psychological trauma: a meta-analysis. *The Lancet, 360,* 766.

Folkman, S., Lazarus, R., Dunkel-Schetter, C., DeLongis, A., & Gruen, R. (1986). Dynamics of a stressful encounter: Cognitive appraisal, coping and encounter outcomes. *Journal of Personality and Social Psychology, 50*(5), 992–1003.

Gist, R. (2001, October). A message of caution. *American Psychological Society Observor.* Available at *www.psychologicalscience.org*

Gist, R., Lohr, J., Kenardy, J., Bergmann, L., Medrum, L., Redburn, B.,

Paton, D., Bisson, J., Woodall, J., & Rosen, G. (1997, May). Researchers speak on CISM. *Emergency Medical Services*, pp. 27–28.

Gist, R., & Woodall, S. T. (2000). There are no simple solutions to complex problems. In J. Violanti, D. Paton, & C. Dunning (Eds.), *Posttraumatic stress intervention: Challenges, issues, and perspectives* (pp. 81–92). Springfield, IL: Charles C. Thomas.

Hokanson, M. (1997, February). Evaluation of the effectiveness of CISM program for the Los Angeles County Fire Department. An applied research project submitted to the National Fire Academy as part of the Executive Fire Officer Program. (Available on interlibrary loan at *www.lrc.fema.gov*)

Kobasa, S. (1979). Stressful life events, personality, and health: An inquire into hardiness. *Journal of Personality and Social Psychology, 37*(1), 1–11.

Larkin, M. (1999, September 18). Can post-traumatic stress disorder be put on hold? *The Lancet, 354*, 1008.

Pennebaker, J. (2000). The effects of traumatic disclosure on physical and mental health: The values of writing and talking about upsetting events. In J. Violanti, D. Paton, & C. Dunning (Eds.), *Posttraumatic stress intervention: Challenges, issues, and perspectives* (pp. 97–111). Springfield, IL: Charles C. Thomas.

Schiess, S. (2000, April). *The effect of critical incident debriefing on the frequency and severity of the symptoms of post traumatic stress disorder.* An applied research project submitted to the National Fire Academy as part of the Executive Fire Officer Program. Available on interlibrary loan at *www.lrc.fema.gov*

Stuhlmiler, C., & Dunning, C. (2000). Challenging the mainstream: From pathogenic to salutogenic models of posttrauma intervention. In J. Violanti, D. Paton, & C. Dunning (Eds.), *Posttraumatic stress intervention: Challenges, issues, and perspectives* (pp. 10–38). Springfield, IL: Charles C. Thomas.

Woodall, J. (1997, January). *Hearts on fire: An ethnographic exploration of the emotional world of firefighters.* Unpublished master's thesis, Ottawa University.

CHAPTER 12

Ackerman, J. (2002, December 18). Firefighters targeted in firehouse arsons: Insurance would build new facility. *Pittsburgh Post-Gazette.*

Al-Anon. (1980). *Are you troubled by someone's drink?* (Available from Al-Anon Family Group Headquarters, Virginia Beach, VA)

Allen, M. (2003, October 15). *Delaware firefighter sues his fire company.* Available at *www.firehouse.com*

Beaton, R. D., & Murphy, S. A. (1995). Working with people in crisis: Research implications. In C. Figley (Ed.), *Compassion fatigue* (pp. 51–81). New York: Brunner/Mazel.

Benson, D. (2002, November 19). Cold brew under fire. *Milwaukee Journal Sentinel.*

Black, R. (2003, November 24). *Alcohol at fire stations under scrutiny.* Available at *www.firehouse.com*

Bleizeffer, D. (2003, June 4). Wyoming fire marshal: Get rid of alcohol. *The Casper Star-Tribune.*

Carter, H. (2003, June 4). *Enough is enough my friends.* Available at *www.firehouse.com*

Cohen, H. C. (2000, February). *Attention-deficit/hyperactivity disorder: Characteristics among emergency medical technicians and firefighters.* Unpublished doctoral dissertation, Walden University.

Estepp, U. J. (1991). Substance abuse. In K. C. Henry & M. D. Shurtleff (Eds.), *Managing people* (Fire Officer Series, Book 1, pp. 141–163). Montgomery, AL: University of Alabama.

Figgins, D. (1990, May). *Does the 24 hour shift cause divorce in the fire service?* An applied research project submitted to the National Fire Academy as part of the Executive Fire Officer Program. (Available on interlibrary loan at *www.lrc.fema.gov*)

Federal Emergency Management Agency. (2003, January). *Firefighter arson: Special report* (USFA-TR-141). (Available at U.S. Fire Administration, 16825 S. Seton Ave., Emmitsburg, MD 21727 or at *www.usfa.fema.gov*)

Flynn, K. (2002, April 6). Fire official will enforce zero tolerance for drug abuse. *New York Times*, Section B, p. 1.

Freedman, A. (1998, September). Camaraderie and organizational dysfunction. *Fire Engineering*, pp. 87–94.

Goode, E. (2002, July 9). Do firefighters like to set fires? *New York Times*, p. 1.

Gottman, J. M., & Silver, N. (1999). *The seven principles for making marriage work.* New York: Crown.

International Association of Fire Chiefs calling for members to adopt new alcohol policy. (2003, September 10). Available at *www.firehouse.com*

Johnson, D., & Murr, A. (2002, July 1). A moth to the flames. *Newsweek*, p. 35.

Lee, H. (2002, September 1). A call to track firefighter arsonists. *San Francisco Chronicle*, p. A23.

MacIntosh, J., & Sheehy, K. (2003, December 1). FDNY wives get burned. *New York Post*, p. 1.

Madigan, N. (2003, December 1). Part-time firefighter is held in setting of blaze in Arizona. *New York Times*.

McGraw, D. K. (1997, May). Is divorce more common in the fire service? Study says no. *Fire Chief*, p. 10.

Murphy, S. A. Bond, G., Beaton, R., Murphy, J., & Johnson, L.C. (2002). Lifestyle practices and occupational stressors as predictors of health outcomes in urban firefighters. *International Journal of Stress Management*, 9(4), 311–327.

North, C. S, Tivis, L., McMillen, J. C., Pfefferbaum, B., Cox, J., Spitznagel, E. L., Bunch, K., Schorr, J., Smith, E. M. (2002). Coping, functioning, and adjustment of rescue workers after the Oklahoma City bombing. *Journal of Traumatic Stress*, 15(3), 171–175.

North, C. S., Tivis, L., McMillen, J. C., Pfefferbaum, B., Spitznagel, E. L., Cox, J., Nixon, S., Bunch, K., & Smith, E. M. (2002). Psychiatric disorders in rescue workers after the Oklahoma City bombing. *American Journal of Psychiatry*, 159, 857–859.

Oregon firefight co. charged with drunk driving. (2003, November 7). Available at *www.firehouse.com*

Shrager, H. (2003, December 2). 9/11 love triangle has deep roots. *Staten Island Advance*, p. 1.

Shrager, H. (2003, December 2). Wife's FDNY Charge: "They Should Have Helped." *Staten Island Advance*, p. 11.

Shrager, H. (2003, December 4). 9/11 couple say their children are being exploited. *Staten Island Advance*, p. 1.

Talbert, J. E. (1996, Febraury). *Divorce in the fire service: A cultural perspective.* An applied research project submitted to the National Fire Academy as part of the Executive Fire Officer Program. (Available on interlibrary loan at *www.lrc.fema.gov*)

Taylor, V., & Wolin, S. (2002). The new normal: How F.D.N.Y. firefighters are rising to the challenge of life after September 11. (Available from the author at *www.2taylors@comcast.net*)

Too close to the fire. (2002, November 20). In *60 Minutes* [TV series]. New York: CBS Broadcasting Inc.

Up front: Are EMTs/paramedics turning to alcohol and drugs to cope with job stress? (1985, January-February). *Emergency Medical Services*, pp. 12–18.

Van Derbeken, J. (2003, November 21). Firefighter says drinking common at S.F. stations. *San Francisco Chronicle*, p. A1.

Wambaugh, J. (2002). *Fire lover.* New York: William Morrow.

CHAPTER 13

Berkman, B., Floren, T., & Willing, L. (1999, November). *Many women strong: A handbook for women firefighters* (USFA EME-5-4651). (Available from Women in the Fire Service, P.O. Box 5446, Madison, WI 53705 or *www.wfis.org*)

Marcucci, P. (2001, June). *When dad is a firefighter: Paternal involvement, parental satisfaction and child's well being.* Unpublished doctoral dissertation, Alliant University.

Woodall, S. J. (1997). Hearts on fire. *Clinical Sociology Review, 15,* 153–162.

CHAPTER 14

Addis, M., & Mahalik, J. (2003, January). Men, masculinity, and the contexts of help seeking. *American Psychologist,* pp. 5–13.

Gottman, J. M. (2001, April). *Clinical manual for marital therapy: A research based approach.* (Available from The Gottman Institute, P.O. Box 15644, Seattle, WA 98115-0644 or *www.gottman.com*)

Gottman, J. M., & Silver, N. (1994). *Why marriages succeed or fail and how you can make yours last.* New York: Simon and Schuster.

Gottman, J. M., & Silver, N. (1999). *The seven principles for making marriage work.* New York: Crown.

Kirschman, E. (1997). *I love a cop: What police families need to know.* New York: Guilford Press.

Index

Index

About the Author

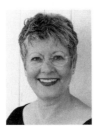

Ellen Kirschman, PhD, is a clinical psychologist, consultant, and public speaker who has been working with fire fighters and police officers and their families for 25 years. She is the author of *I Love a Cop: What Police Families Need to Know* (1997, The Guilford Press).